THE

PET LOVER'S GUIDE TO FIRST AID & EMERGENCIES

About The Pet Lover's Guide Series

Your pets are important members of your family. When they have a medical condition, you want them to get the best care that can be provided. You also want to know everything you can about their condition, including all the treatment options. This series, written by leading veterinary authors, will help you, as a pet owner, understand the causes, diagnosis, treatment, and prevention options for many common conditions your pets may have.

This series provides quality veterinary information, written by the veterinary leaders your veterinarian trusts, but in an easy-to understand manner that allows you to talk with your veterinarian about your pet's condition. **The books in this series are not intended as substitutes for visits to your veterinarian.** Instead, they should be read as a way to get more information about your pet's condition so that you'll know what to do, what to ask, and what to expect when you take your pet to your veterinarian.

THE

PET LOVER'S GUIDE TO FIRST AID & EMERGENCIES

Thomas K. Day

DVM, MS, DACVA, DACVECC

Emergency and Critical Care Veterinarian and
Anesthesiologist
Louisville Veterinary Specialty and
Emergency Services
Louisville, Kentucky

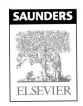

SAUNDERS

ELSEVIER

ELSEVIER
SAUNDERS

11830 Westline Industrial Drive
St. Louis, Missouri 63146

ISBN 13: 978-1-4160-2531-3
ISBN 10: 1-4160-2531-6

The Pet Lover's Guide to First Aid and Emergencies
Copyright © 2006, Elsevier Inc.

The Publisher

ISBN 13: 978-1-4160-2531-3
ISBN 10: 1-4160-2531-6

Publishing Director: Linda Duncan
Acquisitions Editor: Liz Fathman
Developmental Editor: Shelly Stringer
Publishing Services Manager: Patricia Tannian
Project Manager: John Casey
Cover/Book Design Direction: Amy Buxton
Cover/Book Design: Bill Smith Studio

Printed in United States of America

Last digit is the print number: 9   8   7   6   5   4   3   2   1

For my beautiful Halle

Your short time here inspired us to
love life and each other
unconditionally

Acknowledgments

I would like to thank the staff of Louisville Veterinary Specialty and Emergency Services for their assistance.

I would also like to thank the pet owners who gave their permission to allow pictures of their pets to be published in this book.

Introduction

The Pet Lover's Guide to First Aid and Emergencies starts by describing what is normal and expected in your pet and then moves into descriptions of the most common emergency situations in dogs and cats. Instead of talking about a specific diagnosis, however, the emphasis is on the clinical signs in dogs and cats, like limping or difficulty breathing. The related emergency problems of dogs and cats are discussed as they relate to each clinical sign. Clinical signs are described in three distinct categories based on the concept of "triage," the method used by both human and veterinary emergency hospitals to determine which patients require more immediate attention. Using the table of contents, you, the pet owner, can find the clinical sign (such as burns or snakebite) and then find the chapter to determine the severity of the emergency. Each chapter provides information on first aid do's and don'ts for the particular emergency and covers dogs and cats. The book also describes cardiopulmonary resuscitation (CPR) and also provides suggestions for a pet first aid kit, including lists of which human drugs can be given to pets and which should not be. Text boxes entitled "Where We Stand" are included to provide you, the pet owner, with the professional opinion of the author regarding specific issues in first aid and emergencies.

This book is not a substitute for professional help. It should be used in emergencies and only until the client can take the pet into the veterinarian or emergency clinic, as needed. Of course, some emergencies are minor and do not require a trip to the veterinarian, and when that is the case, the book is an effective guide for watchful waiting.

Contents

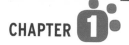

INTRODUCTION TO PET FIRST AID

What Is an Emergency?

Pets are considered a part of the family. Pet owners are very observant and concerned when it comes to the health of their pets.

When a pet is ill or injured, pet owners want to have some idea of whether veterinary attention is required. Regardless of the excellent training of veterinary emergency hospital reception staff or the excellent care provided by the veterinarian *after* the pet is brought for treatment, it will be you as the pet owner who initially observes the ill or injured animal. So it will be up to you to decide whether or not the problem is an emergency. Many emergencies occur at night and on weekends, when your veterinarian may not be on duty to assist you in making a decision.

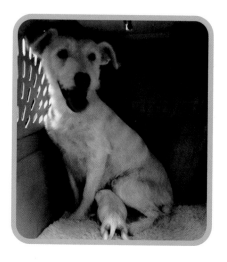

A firm definition of an emergency is very difficult to pinpoint. But as a rule, if you feel that your pet requires veterinary attention, you should seek veterinary attention.

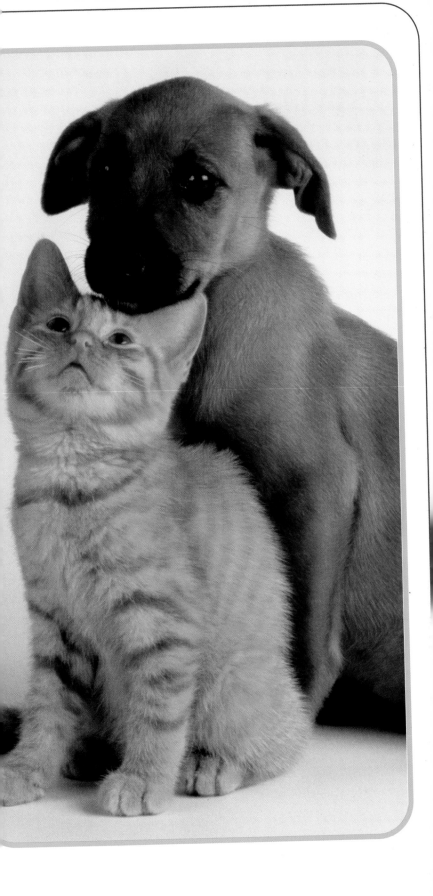

How Can Pet Owners Provide First Aid?

Once an emergency situation has been determined, a decision must be made about the first aid needs of the pet.

Pet owners can provide life-saving first aid in many cases. This book can help guide you in determining what can be done until the pet is brought to the veterinary emergency hospital.

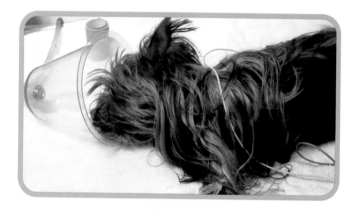

When you see a dog or a cat that has been injured and requires immediate attention, you may want to help even though the animal is not your pet. First aid is required in most of these cases as well. Most veterinary emergency hospitals will accept and treat injured dogs and cats brought in by Good Samaritans.

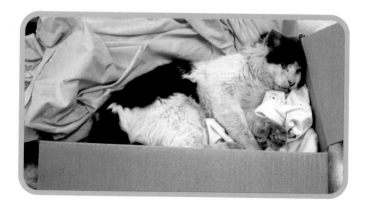

How Can Pet Owners Use This Book?

This book describes the most common emergency situations in dogs and cats. Rarely can anyone tell what the diagnosis is at the time of the emergency. Therefore, the emphasis of the book is on the clinical medical signs that can be observed in the ill or injured animal, rather than on the actual cause of these abnormalities. For example, in this book the clinical sign of "difficulty breathing" will be discussed instead of a specific diagnosis of asthma or congestive heart failure or collapsed lung from a chest injury (any of which may cause difficulty breathing).

Emergency problems of dogs and of cats are discussed for each clinical sign.

Clinical signs are described in three distinct categories based on the concept of **triage** (in which injuries or illnesses are classified as critical, less serious, or minor). Triage is used in human and veterinary emergency hospitals to determine which patients require more immediate attention. (Chapter 3 includes a detailed discussion of triage.) In this book, you will find specific recommendations for life-saving first aid measures and stabilization techniques that you can apply until you can get your pet to a veterinarian.

"Where We Stand" Boxes

This book contains a lot of information, with many illustrations and photographs. Ready access to certain basics is important, however, because emergency situations can require immediate decisions regarding first aid.

Throughout the book, "Where We Stand" boxes highlight the professional opinion of the author regarding important points in first aid for pets. You can refer to the "Where We Stand" information to quickly identify key steps to take and mistakes to avoid in a specific emergency situation.

First Aid versus Therapy

Many concepts of first aid for pets presented in this book have been adopted from human emergency medicine practice. Emergency medical technicians—paramedics—are highly trained and follow protocols created by

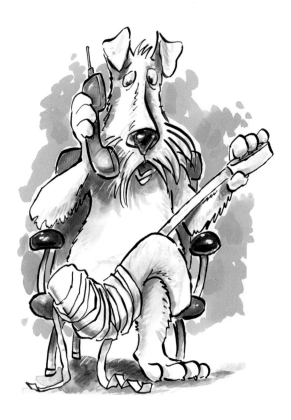

physicians who are specialists in emergency medicine. Paramedics do not act without permission provided directly from established policies or instructions by the physician at the hospital.

Pet owners are not trained to provide specific therapy in emergency situations. This book can help you provide safe and effective first aid to injured and ill dogs and cats, but it is *not* to be used as a manual of definitive care.

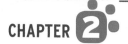

CHAPTER 2

THE NORMAL PET DOG AND CAT

You will need to know and understand what "normal" is before you can decide whether **first aid** is needed and what first aid to give. This chapter reviews what is considered normal body function in dogs and cats, grouped into four main areas:

- Alertness
- Airway
- Breathing
- Circulation

These categories also form the backbone of the **ABC principle** of first aid, covered in Chapter 3.

Where We Stand

We feel that the pet owner should determine normal parameters for the pet. The pet owner can use this knowledge to determine abnormalities sooner. Any deviation from normal could be an emergency situation.

Normal Mental Alertness and Behavior

Pet owners know the level of mental alertness and behavior of their dog or cat very well. Any change from normal could indicate an emergency situation.

6

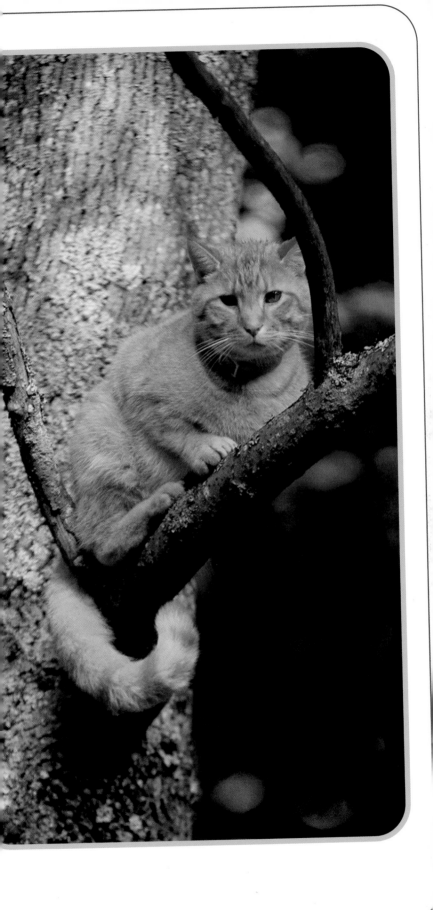

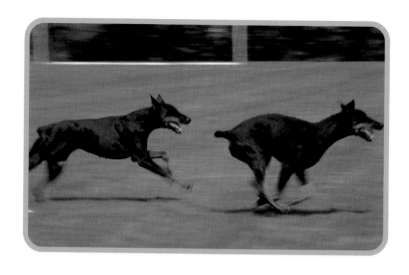

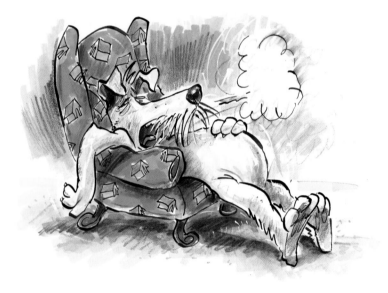

Normal Airway

The normal dog and cat should breathe at rest with the mouth closed and without a lot of noise.

Dogs with "flat faces" (**brachycephalic** breeds, such as the Bulldog, Boston Terrier, Pug, and Pekingese) commonly make snorting or snoring sounds when breathing in with the mouth closed, especially during sleep.

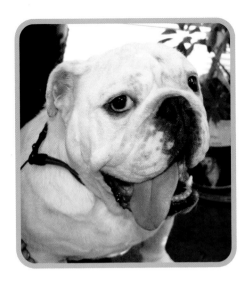

Cats with "flat faces," such as the Himalayan and Persian, typically do not make snoring sounds. But the owner may hear louder *breath* sounds.

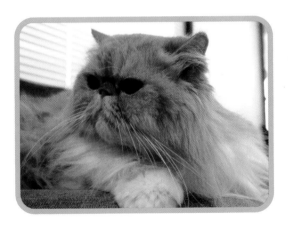

Normal Breathing

Normal breaths or respirations occur without much effort.

Inspiration (breathing in) is an active process and is seen as an upward or outward movement of the chest. This movement should occur easily with the mouth closed. The muscles of the face or nose should not move much.

Expiration (breathing out) is entirely passive. When your pet is at rest, the abdominal muscles should not move much, as they might when your pet is grunting. The abdominal muscles will be involved with expiration only when your pet is exercising.

In other words, your pet's chest should rise and fall without effort while it is at rest.

The *normal breathing rate* at rest for dogs depends somewhat on the size of the animal:

- **Small or toy breeds (Poodle, Chihuahua, Yorkshire Terrier):** 15 to 30 breaths per minute at rest
- **Medium breeds (Australian Shepherd, Boxer):** 10 to 25 breaths per minute at rest
- **Large breeds (Labrador Retriever, German Shepherd Dog, Golden Retriever):** 10 to 20 breaths per minute at rest
- **Giant breeds (Great Dane, Irish Wolfhound, Malamute):** 8 to 20 breaths per minute at rest

Normal dogs can pant up to 200 breaths per minute after exercise or in warm temperatures. Puppies and kittens up to 8 to 10 weeks of age breathe at a rate of 60 to 100 breaths per minute at rest.

The normal breathing rate in the cat is 20 to 40 breaths per minute at rest. Cats do not pant. Panting in a cat is a sign of a serious problem.

Normal Circulation

The Complex Nature of Blood Circulation

The body must circulate blood to provide enough oxygen to all tissues. You can tell how well this complex process is working by measuring the heart rate and rhythm, pulse rate and strength, and coordination of heart and pulse rates—the **circulation parameters.** You can easily figure out the basic circulation parameters of heart rate and pulse rate, as discussed next. Remember that an abnormality in one parameter, like pulse rate, will result in an abnormality in another parameter, like heart rate. If the underlying problem gets worse, your pet may show signs of depression or be lethargic.

Other ways you can assess the function of the circulation are by looking at the color of the gums and other mucous membranes and measuring **capillary refill time.**

Heart Rate

The heart rate can be found by placing your hands on either side of the chest (in medium to large dogs) or by cupping one hand over the central part of the chest (in small dogs and cats), just behind the elbow of the front legs.

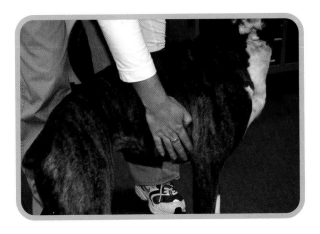

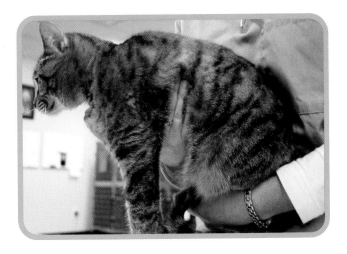

The *normal heart rate* at rest for dogs depends somewhat on the size of the animal:

- **Small or toy breeds (Poodle, Chihuahua, Yorkshire Terrier):** 80 to 120 beats per minutes at rest
- **Medium breeds (Australian Shepherd, Boxer):** 60 to 120 beats per minute at rest
- **Large breeds (Labrador Retriever, German Shepherd Dog, Golden Retriever):** 60 to 110 beats per minutes at rest
- **Giant breeds (Great Dane, Irish Wolfhound, Malamute):** 50 to 100 beats per minute at rest

Athletic dogs will have somewhat lower heart rates than those listed. Puppies and kittens up to the age of 8 to 10 weeks have a heart rate between 150 and 200 beats per minute.

The normal heart rate for cats is 160 to 200 beats per minute.

Pulse Rate

The pulse rate is most easily felt in the femoral artery. The femoral artery is located on the inside of the rear leg near the abdomen. Place your left hand under the left rear leg as you approach from the front of the leg with your thumb located on the outside of the leg and your four fingers on the inside of the leg. You can do the same thing

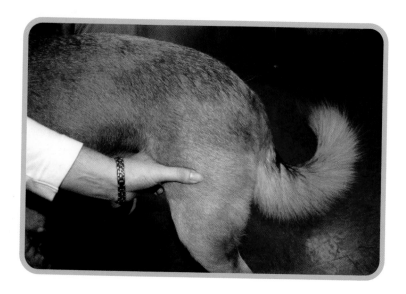

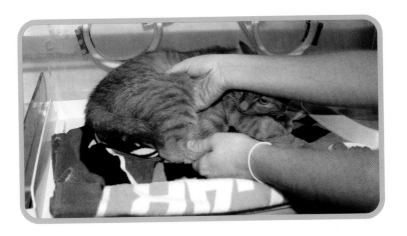

with the right hand using the right rear leg. Make certain that your hands are as close to the abdomen as possible. The femoral artery is located just in front of the femur bone. Lightly feel the pulse (the pulsation of the artery) with the tips of your index, middle, and ring fingers.

Finding the pulse is easiest in a large, thin dog such as a Greyhound. The pulse is harder to find in an animal that is lying down than in an animal that is standing. The pulse is hardest to find in cats and obese dogs.

Coordination of Heart Rate and Pulse Rate

The pulse rate should be the same as the heart rate.

The pulse will be felt a split second after the heartbeat occurs, as the femoral artery is located far enough away from the heart to make a difference in timing of the two.

Alternative Locations to Feel the Pulse

Another useful artery is located on the underside of the front paw, and the pulse in this artery can be felt most easily in medium- and larger-breed dogs. It is difficult to feel in cats and small dogs.

An extension of the femoral artery runs along the inside of the rear leg between the toes and the heel. Again, the pulse in this artery can be felt most easily in medium- and larger-breed dogs and is very difficult to feel in cats and small dogs.

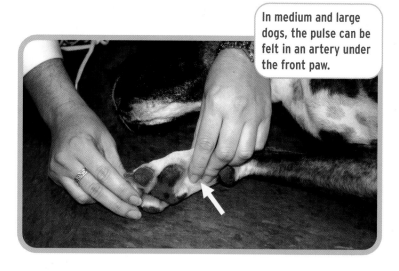

In medium and large dogs, the pulse can be felt in an artery under the front paw.

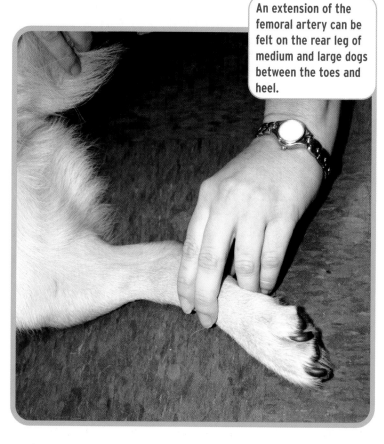

An extension of the femoral artery can be felt on the rear leg of medium and large dogs between the toes and heel.

The artery located in the ear of the Bassett Hound can be palpated on the outside of the ear near its center.

Occasionally, the artery located under the base of the tail can be felt in breeds of dogs with short hair coats.

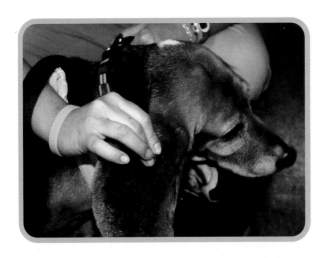

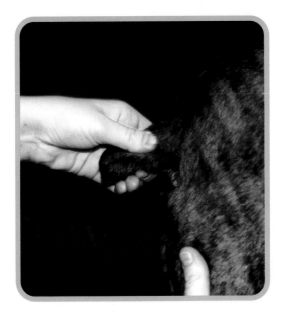

Gum (Mucous Membrane) Color and Capillary Refill Time

The mucous membranes contain a high concentration of blood vessels. The gums are the easiest location to use in looking at mucous membrane color, which can give you an idea about the amount of blood flow to the gums.

Capillary refill refers to the amount of time it takes the gums (or other mucous membranes) to return to normal color after they are gently compressed with a finger or thumb.

Normal Gum Color

The normal gum color in dogs and cats is light pink.

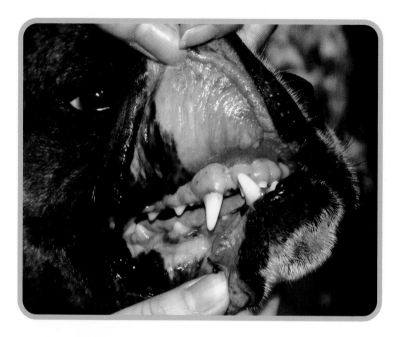

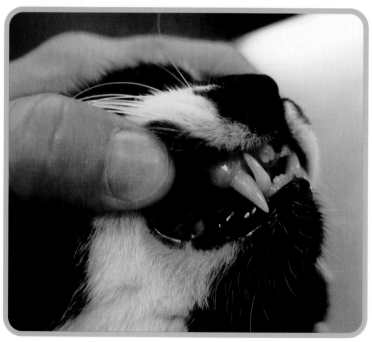

Some dogs have normal black pigment on the gums and the inside of the lips. Assessing the gum color may be difficult in these dogs.

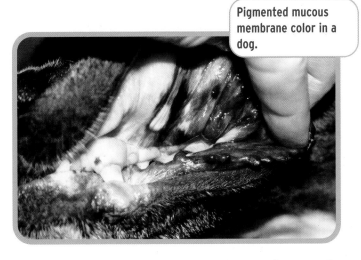

Pigmented mucous membrane color in a dog.

Cats and small dogs have a relatively smaller area in the mouth to examine gum color, making assessment more difficult.

Alternative Sites to Assess Mucous Membrane Color

Dogs

- The inside lining of the eyelids
- The inside lining of the rectum

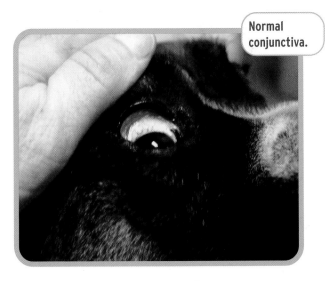

Normal conjunctiva.

Male dog

- The inside tips of the prepuce (or foreskin), especially in dogs with a large amount of black pigment of the gums

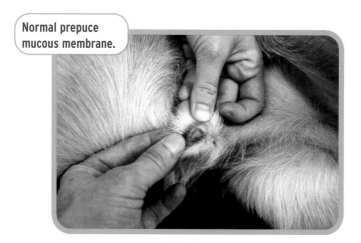

Normal prepuce mucous membrane.

Female dog

- The inside of the vulvar tissue, especially in dogs with a large amount of black pigment of the gums

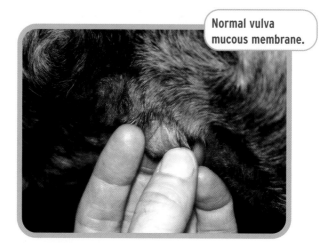

Normal vulva mucous membrane.

Cat

- The inside lining of the eyelids (the only feasible alternative location to assess mucous membrane color in cats)

Normal Capillary Refill Time

Gently compressing an area of the gums with your thumb, as you hold the lip out of the way, should result in a temporary blanching (whitening) of the tissue. This effect is seen as the blood is pressed out of the small blood vessels called capillaries. When your thumb is released, the white spot where your thumb applied pressure should then turn back to light pink within 1 to 2 seconds. This is called the **capillary refill time.**

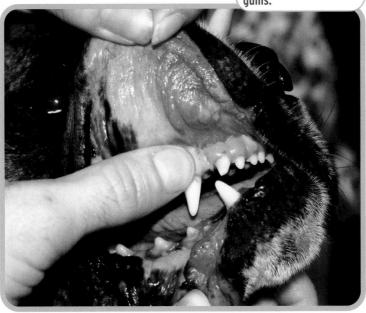

Capillary refill time can help you determine how effectively the heart and blood vessels provide enough blood to the tissue.

Normal Rectal Body Temperature

Body temperature in dogs and cats is measured with a rectal thermometer. The digital thermometers most people use with children are more accurate than mercury thermometers. Digital thermometers can measure the higher body temperatures that normally occur in dogs and cats.

Lubricate the thermometer with petroleum jelly and gently insert the end of the thermometer approximately 1 inch into the rectum. Digital thermometers display the temperature within 30 to 60 seconds.

Normal rectal body temperature in dogs and cats ranges from approximately 100 to 102.5 degrees Fahrenheit.

CHAPTER 3

RECOGNIZING AN EMERGENCY

To recognize an emergency situation, you will need to be familiar with normal physical findings in dogs and cats (as described in Chapter 2). Then you will need to closely examine your pet for any signs of *life-threatening* problems. Use the **ABC principle**—Alertness and Airway, Breathing, and Circulation—to do a quick assessment.

The **RAP principle,** similar to the ABC principle, also can be used for a quick assessment. With this approach, the areas of assessment are Respiration (breathing), Alertness, and Perfusion (blood circulation).

Abnormal Mental Alertness and Behavior

The first change you may notice in your pet is a decrease in mental awareness (depression or lethargy) or a difference from its usual behavior.

A common clinical sign in pets brought to the emergency hospital, which can occur either alone or in combination with other clinical signs, is depression or lethargy. When your pet shows signs of depression or lethargy, it may be unable to walk, get tired after mild or moderate exercise, be reluctant to move, hang its head, and hold its tail between its legs. A common sign of depression in the cat is excessive sleeping and difficulty waking when asleep, even with other activity in the room.

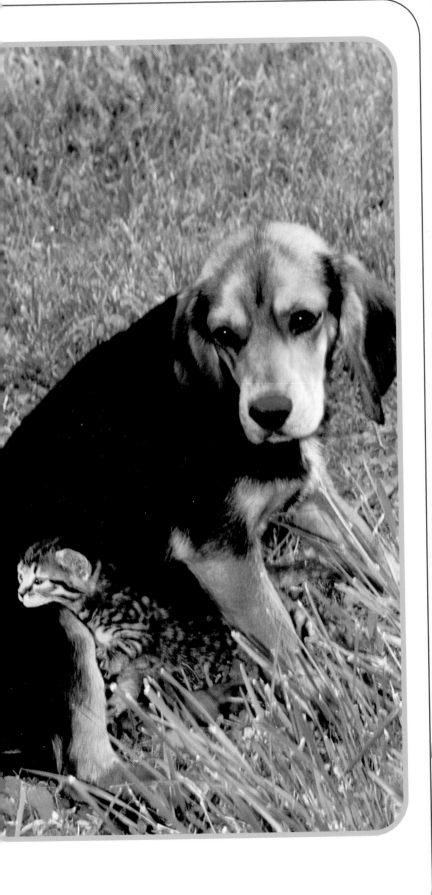

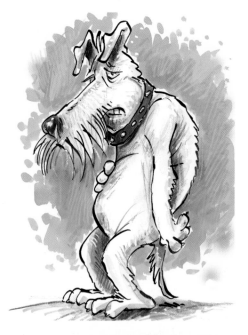

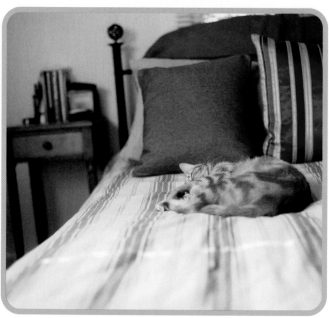

On the other hand, you may observe excitement in your pet, rather than depression. Your pet may become excited if it swallows certain over-the-counter and prescription medications, chocolate, nicotine, and some herbicides or pesticides.

Aggressive or submissive behavior in dogs and cats may be a signal that they are in pain, especially in cats.

Abnormal Airway

Dogs and cats that are not brachycephalic (flat-faced) breeds should not have noisy breathing with the mouth closed or open.

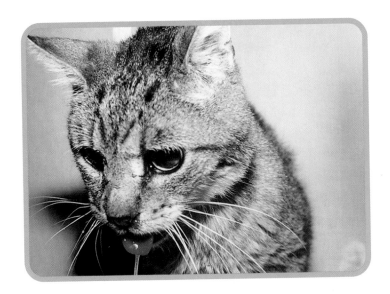

A dog or cat that you can hear breathing may have a serious upper airway problem such as obstruction by a foreign object, a mass such as a tumor, or general swelling of the throat.

Abnormal Breathing

If your pet uses increased effort on inspiration (breathing in) and/or expiration (breathing out), it signals an immediate emergency, especially if the dog or cat is breathing with the mouth open.

Less obvious changes can occur in dogs and cats with respiratory problems. For example, you may notice an increase in breathing *rate* without an increase in breathing *effort*. Cats with respiratory problems can have an increased breathing rate before they show signs of increased breathing effort.

Abnormal Circulation Parameters

If your pet has abnormalities in its circulation, usually it will show signs of changes in more than one circulation parameter. For example, changes in mucous membrane color, **capillary refill time,** and heart and pulse rates may all occur at the same time.

Heart Rate

Your pet's heart rate can be abnormally high or abnormally low. However, it is difficult to provide solid guidelines for determining what is too high and what is too low. Knowing your pet's normal heart rate will help you determine whether it is too high or too low.

Most dogs and cats that have heart rates that are too high or too low also have changes in mental alertness, mucous membrane color, and capillary refill time.

Pulse Rate

Your pet's pulse rate and strength of the pulse can also be too fast or too slow. The pulse also can be weaker than normal or may vary in its intensity.

Coordination of Heart Rate and Pulse Rate

If there is an abnormality, the pulse rate is usually slower than the heart rate when you feel both at the same time. Typically, a high heart rate with a lower pulse rate indicates a potential emergency.

Gum (Mucous Membrane) Color

When your pet's blood pressure decreases, its mucous membranes may become pale, gray, or white. This is usually accompanied by either a high or an extremely low heart rate.

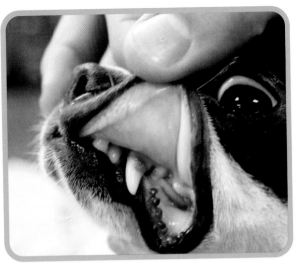

Pale, gray, or white mucous membranes also can indicate a decrease in the number of red blood cells.

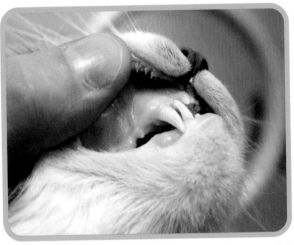

When the mucous membranes are blue (cyanosis), it indicates your pet is not getting enough oxygen.

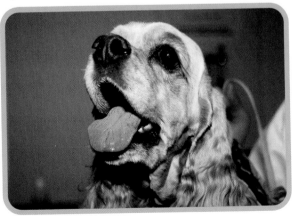

Brown mucous membranes in cats are usually a sign of acetaminophen (Tylenol) poisoning.

Yellow mucous membranes (jaundice) indicate either a liver disorder or a red blood cell problem.

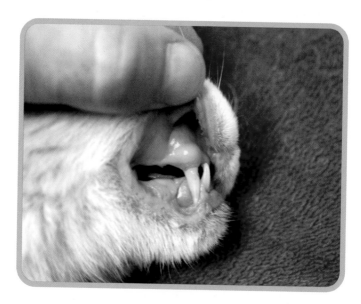

Mucous membranes can also be too pink. Bright red or brick red mucous membranes can tell you that there is infection somewhere in your pet's body.

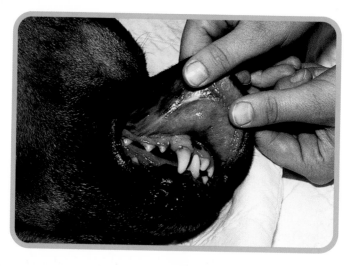

Capillary Refill Time

An increase in the time it takes to return the gums to normal color, after you have blanched them (by applying pressure to them with your thumb and finger—see

Chapter 2 for more information about capillary refill time), indicates poor blood flow. If the capillary refill time is greater than 2 seconds, your pet should be examined by a veterinarian.

An increase in capillary refill time is usually associated with either a high or an extremely low heart rate.

When your pet's mucous membranes are very pale or white, indicating poor blood flow, you may not be able to determine capillary refill time.

The capillary refill time can be shorter than normal in dogs with bright or brick red mucous membranes. A capillary refill time less than 1 second in a dog with bright red mucous membranes indicates an abnormality.

Where We Stand

We feel that a pet with any abnormality in alertness, airway, breathing, or circulation requires immediate first aid and should be taken to a veterinary hospital.

The Concept of Triage

Abnormalities in breathing and/or circulation parameters may indicate an emergency.

Human and veterinary emergency hospitals use the concept of **triage** to help determine which patients require more immediate attention. Triage is the process of prioritizing sick or injured people or animals for treatment. The patient is assigned to one of three categories of decreasing severity—according to whether the illness or injury is critical, less serious, or minor.

You can decide whether your pet needs immediate veterinary attention by using the concept of triage. The

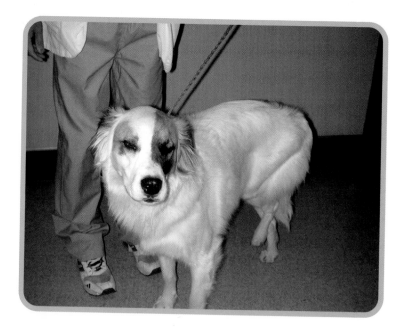

triage level also can determine the need for and the type of **first aid.**

The three levels of triage used in clinical veterinary emergency practice are:

Triage Level 1: The illness or injury is critical, and the pet may survive if simple life-saving measures are applied.

Triage Level 2: The pet is likely to survive if simple care is given within hours.

Triage Level 3: The pet has minor injuries, so care can be delayed while other patients with more critical injuries are treated.

Pet Owners' Use of Triage

Pet owners can use the general guidelines of triage to determine the immediate first aid needs of their ill or injured dog and cat.

Obvious Emergencies—Based on Triage Levels 1 and 2

- **Any change in alertness, airway, breathing, or circulation means that your pet needs immediate veterinary attention.**

- First aid usually is required in these pets.
- Specific first aid measures that can be applied by pet owners for pets assigned triage levels 1 and 2 are covered in Chapters 6 and 7.

Less Urgent Problems—Based on Triage Level 3

- Many illnesses or injuries that are not immediately life-threatening will require some sort of first aid.
- Specific first aid that can be applied by pet owners for pets assigned triage level 3 is covered in Chapter 8.
- Pet owners must understand that first aid is not definitive care. Only your veterinarian can provide specific care for the pet.

CHAPTER 4

APPROACH TO FIRST AID

Definition of First Aid

First aid is the use of basic treatment techniques at the scene of an accident or in cases of sudden severe illness. It is similar to the care provided by "first responders" in human emergency medicine. More advanced care (such as setting a broken bone or giving medication for a severe infection) by the first aid provider is not expected and is best left to the veterinarian. In life-threatening emergencies, however, pet owners can apply lifesaving treatment using the first aid techniques described in this book (see Chapters 6 to 8).

Safety

Ensure your own safety. As the person performing first aid, this is your first responsibility. Injured or severely ill animals can act unpredictably during handling, even toward a person trying to help them. Not concerned for

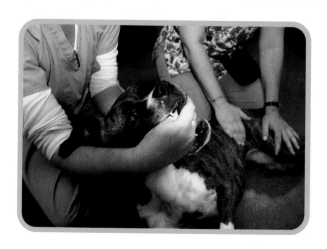

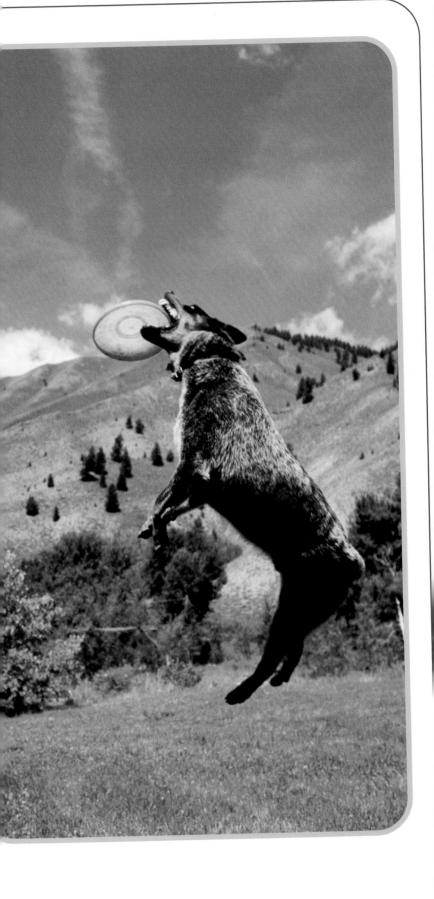

your own safety? Keep in mind that if you *are* bitten or scratched, you may then be unable to help the animal needing your aid.

Evaluate the situation and setting. A busy roadway is a dangerous place for both the injured animal and yourself. "Safety first" is the key, even when the danger to the animal seems to be increasing (as when an injured dog runs onto the highway). Take the situation and any potential dangers into account, and act appropriately to keep yourself and those around you safe.

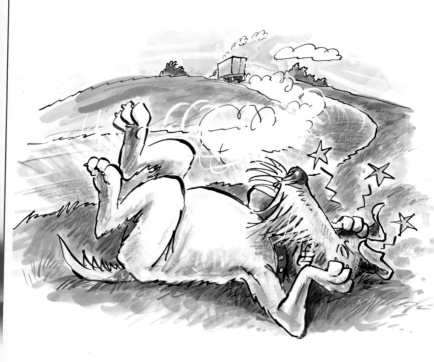

Do No Harm

Restrain the ill or injured animal carefully. Your goal in an emergency setting is to provide aid but to **do no harm**. Incorrect or aggressive handling could be harmful to the animal.

Do not give medication without a veterinarian's recommendation. Even common over-the-counter medications

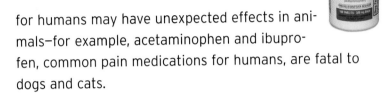

for humans may have unexpected effects in animals—for example, acetaminophen and ibuprofen, common pain medications for humans, are fatal to dogs and cats.

Why Is Restraint Necessary?

Use of **restraint** techniques is almost always recommended for the injured dog or cat, whether it is a pet of yours or a stray animal.

Even the most gentle or docile dog or cat can behave unpredictably and violently when injured.

Injured animals that appear docile may not remain docile when they are given first aid, even in the owner's presence (for example, when direct pressure is applied to a bleeding wound).

Remember, your safety is the first priority. The main reason to restrain an injured animal is to prevent unintentional harm to you during first aid.

Restraint Techniques

Muzzles

Use a muzzle to prevent the injured animal from biting you.

Applying a muzzle on long-nosed dogs is easier than in shorter-nosed dogs and in most cats.

Improvise a muzzle: A variety of materials can be used to make a muzzle, including rope, towels, and T-shirts. Make a loose half-knot under the bottom jaw, and extend and tie a square knot behind the animal's head.

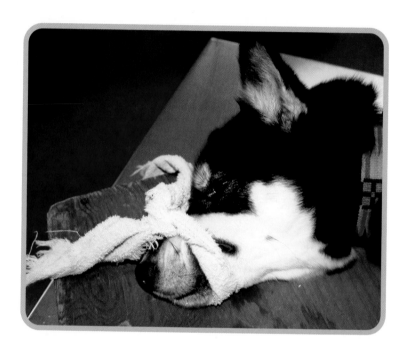

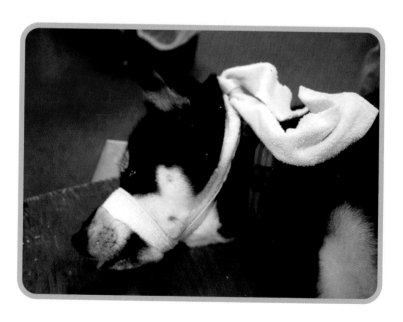

Commercially made muzzles for dogs are preferable to homemade ones, as they are more effective in preventing biting.

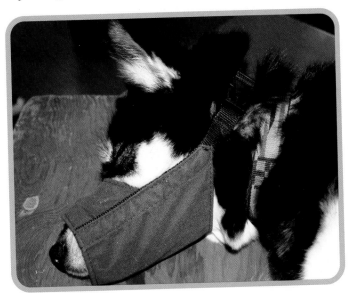

Be careful when placing a commercially made muzzle on a cat, especially a stray cat. These muzzles tend to cover the entire face. Cats typically do not like this feeling and may begin to struggle even more.

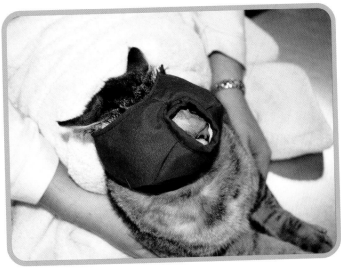

The animal should be able to open its mouth to breathe with the muzzle on. The goal is not to completely close the mouth, but to keep the mouth closed enough to prevent biting.

Do not use a muzzle on animals that are having difficulty breathing.

Towels and Blankets

Large towels or blankets can be used to restrain most cats and small dogs.

Place the entire thick towel or blanket over and snugly around the animal so that you can handle and transport the animal without being injured.

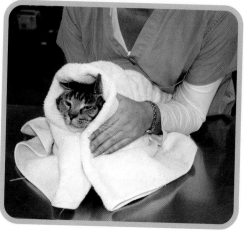

Be very careful when handling animals that are having difficulty breathing. Use minimal restraint.

Fishnets and other netting devices can be used to safely capture and restrain stray cats.

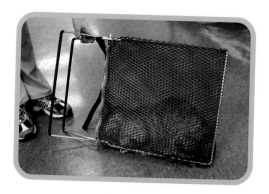

Physical Restraint

When handling injured cats, use a firm grasp of the scruff of the neck and the hind legs if you can't use a blanket, towel, or net.

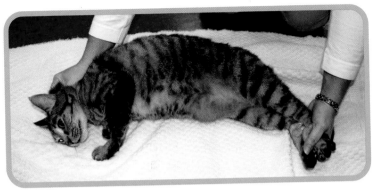

Small dogs can be physically restrained with the towel or blanket technique.

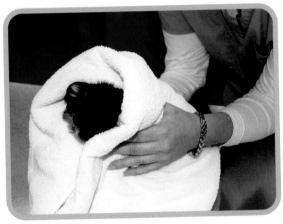

You may need to physically restrain medium and large dogs. In this case, place one arm under the dog's neck, using your hand to secure the back of the dog's head. Place your second arm over the dog's chest, using your other hand to secure the dog's lower chest. You may need assistance in restraining the dog's hind legs. As always, your safety is the primary consideration.

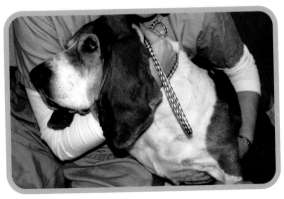

Restraint Techniques That Are Not Recommended

Hobbles are not recommended, especially if you think your pet might have a broken bone.

Never tie all four of the limbs together.

Be careful when tying anything around the neck. Do not tie half-knots or square knots, as they tighten too easily.

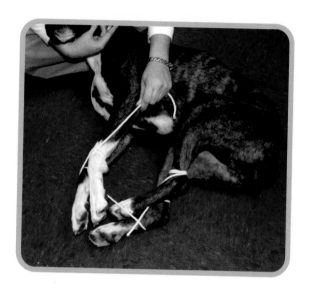

Transport

The best thing you can do for an ill or injured animal is to take it to a veterinary clinic or hospital.

Make sure to ensure your safety during transport.

Take care to prevent further injury to the animal during transport.

Leave the injured animal alone during transport, because further restraint often causes more stress. Even the pet's owner should avoid handling the pet during transport.

Make the animal as comfortable as possible.

Take special care in transporting stray dogs and cats. Stray animals usually are wary of people, and an injured stray may become frightened when it is approached.

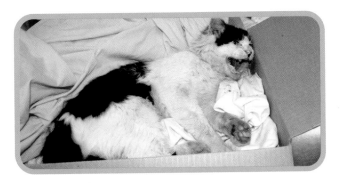

Stray cats can be especially difficult to transport. Restrain an injured stray cat with a blanket or towel, and place the cat, uncovered, in a towel-lined box. When possible, use a net for capturing especially difficult cats.

Transport of medium and large dogs is challenging. Larger dogs are difficult to lift and place in a vehicle, and injured dogs may be even more difficult to move safely.

Use a piece of plywood or other solid surface as a makeshift stretcher for transport. Secure the injured dog to the surface with tape or rope.

Secure the injured dog or cat safely when you are transporting it in the bed of a truck or other uncovered vehicle.

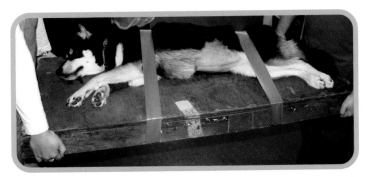

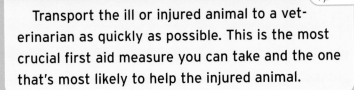

Where We Stand

Transport the ill or injured animal to a veterinarian as quickly as possible. This is the most crucial first aid measure you can take and the one that's most likely to help the injured animal.

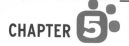

CHAPTER 5

CARDIOPULMONARY-CEREBRAL RESUSCITATION (CPCR) IN PETS

Definitions

Cardiopulmonary-Cerebral Resuscitation (CPCR)

You've probably seen or heard the term **cardiopulmonary resuscitation** (CPR). This term is used to describe a technique to revive (resuscitate) people or animals when they are unconscious or appear to be dead. CPR uses techniques that temporarily replace or imitate functions of the heart and the lungs (together these are called **cardiopulmonary function**).

Where We Stand

Even when performed by prepared first aid providers, CPCR will not be enough to protect the brain and prevent death. A physical examination and further emergency treatment by a veterinarian are necessary, even if the CPCR is successful.

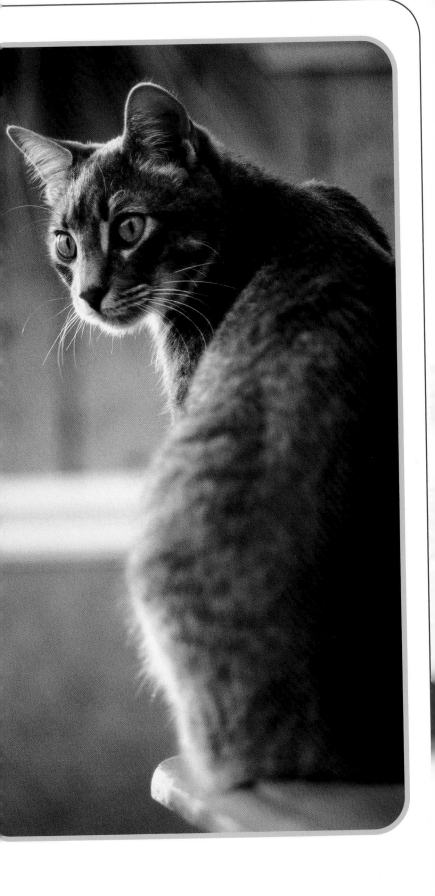

We also know that although the heart and lungs can be returned to normal function with CPR, the pet still may not survive because the brain dies. So restoring brain (cerebral) function is considered a vital step in revival or resuscitation. Together, restoration of normal heart, lung, and brain function is known as CPCR.

Death (Arrest)

Signs of death, or arrest (that is, when vital body functions appear to stop), must be clearly present before CPCR should be attempted.

The medical or clinical definition of death includes one or more of the following:

- **Breathing has completely stopped.**
- **No heartbeat or pulse can be felt on palpation (feeling with the fingers).**
- **Blue (cyanotic) gums remain blue.**
- **Unconsciousness cannot be restored.**

Of course it is possible for an unconscious animal to still be breathing and have a heartbeat and pulse. A nasty bite may be the result of attempting to perform CPR on an animal that suddenly regains consciousness!

Respiratory Arrest vs. Cardiac Arrest

It is very important for you, as the pet first aid provider, to understand the difference between *respiratory* arrest and *cardiac* arrest. That way you can administer CPCR most effectively.

The primary cause of death in animals is **respiratory arrest,** or a total inability to continue breathing. Most life-threatening diseases and injuries of pets happen when the brain can no longer tell the lungs to breathe.

On the other hand, the primary cause of death in *people* is **cardiac arrest.** When the coronary arteries become blocked, heart beats become irregular and heart muscles die from lack of oxygen (called myocardial infarction or heart attack). Heart function usually stops before lung and brain functions do.

Coronary artery disease is rare in dogs and has so far not been seen in cats.

Heart disease in dogs and cats causes the lungs to work less efficiently, and usually breathing stops before heart circulation stops (cardiac arrest).

Basic Life Support CPCR (BLS CPCR)

Basic life support (BLS) measures should be started when there are obvious clinical signs of arrest (as described below) and the pet is unconscious:

- **Breathing has stopped.**
- **No heart rate or pulse can be felt.**
- **Gums are blue.**

BLS follows the **ABC principle** discussed in Chapter 3 (Recognizing an Emergency)

Airway

- **Your pet's airway must be cleared before you start to deliver breaths.**
- **Dogs and cats cannot swallow their tongues!**
- **Make sure your pet is unconscious and that the mouth can be opened easily and without resistance.**
- **Remember: your safety comes first!**

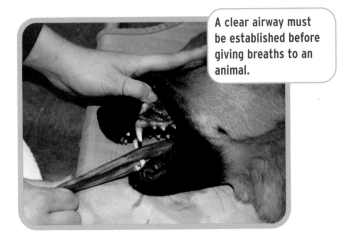

A clear airway must be established before giving breaths to an animal.

Breathing

■ Use one hand to close your pet's mouth to make sure no air escapes during your breath. Using the other hand, gently apply pressure to both sides of the windpipe (trachea) to prevent your breath from entering the stomach instead of the lungs.

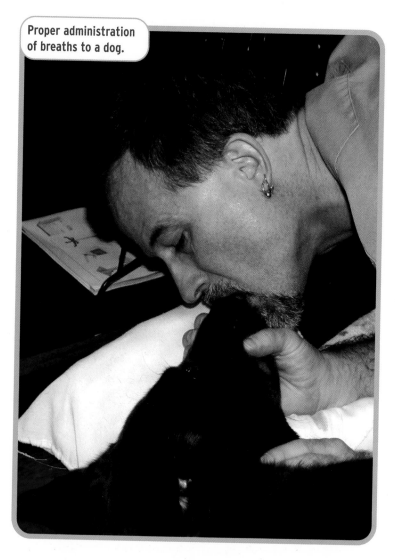

Proper administration of breaths to a dog.

■ Gently breathe from your mouth into your pet's nostrils for no longer than 1 to 1.5 seconds per breath.
■ The smaller the dog, and always with cats, the more gentle the breaths.

The normal rate of breathing should be between 15 and 20 breaths per minute in both dogs and cats.

44

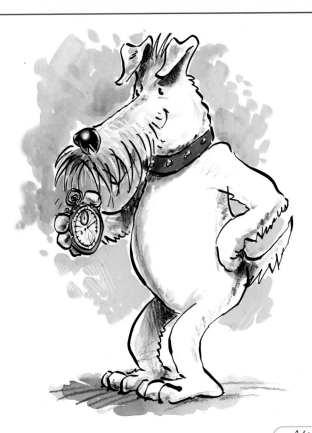

Three common mistakes in giving artificial respiration are:

- Breathing too hard, which can damage the lungs
- Breathing air into the stomach instead of the lungs
- Breathing too fast

Circulation

You provide artificial circulation by pressing on the chest (chest compressions).

- ■ **Caution:** Pets with obvious chest injury should not be given chest compressions.

Your goal is to provide enough blood flow to the brain and heart to restore sufficient function. Note, however, that chest compressions alone will not provide *normal* blood flow to the brain.

Depending on the number of first aid providers present to perform CPCR and the size of your pet, there are two different techniques for performing chest compressions.

- ■ **One person can successfully perform CPCR, but two people are ideal. When only one person is providing CPCR, the focus should be on providing adequate breaths to the pet. Provide two consecutive breaths followed by five consecutive chest compressions, and continue to repeat.**
- ■ **When two people are performing CPCR, one person concentrates on providing 15 to 20 breaths per minute. The second person provides chest compressions, as described next, at a rate of 100 compressions per minute.**

Small Dogs and Cats (100 Compressions per Minute)

- ■ **One or both hands can be placed around the bottom or top of the chest when the pet is lying on its side.**
- ■ **Deliver all compressions to the middle of the chest or ribcage, not necessarily over the heart.**

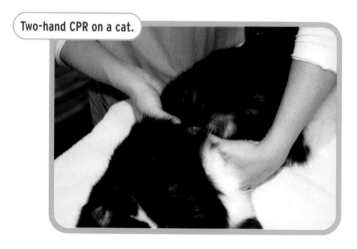

Two-hand CPR on a cat.

- ■ **Focus the compressions to a single spot. Ribs can easily be broken. The heat of the moment may find you providing too vigorous chest compressions!**

Medium and Large Dogs (100 Compressions per Minute)

- Place your pet on its side and position yourself with your pet's back toward you. You may use your legs or thighs to keep your pet from moving during compressions.
- Straighten your arms, interlock the fingers of both hands together, and place your hands on the widest portion of the chest. Remember: Direct compressions over the heart will not be as effective as compressions over the widest part of the chest.

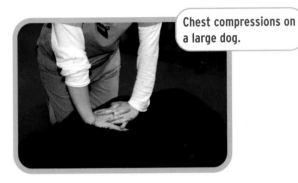

Chest compressions on a large dog.

- Begin compressions at 100 compressions per minute.
- Do not compress more than half of the width of the chest. Ribs can easily be broken. The heat of the moment may find you providing too vigorous chest compressions!
- Performing one-person CPCR on a large dog is challenging. For best results, get additional help if at all possible.

Advanced Life Support CPCR (ALS CPCR)

Advanced life support (ALS) is intended to restore blood flow to the brain as well as to provide basic resuscitation.

ALS can be performed only in a veterinary hospital.

ALS consists of giving specific drugs and medications, in addition to providing continual artificial breaths with a respirator. Surgery may be necessary in some instances, especially when traumatic injuries are involved.

Immediate transport to a veterinary hospital is essential.

BLS may be required during transport.

CHAPTER 6

FIRST AID FOR TRIAGE LEVEL 1 PATIENTS

Definition

With triage level 1, a pet's injury or illness is critical, but the pet may survive if simple lifesaving steps are taken. Immediate first aid and veterinary attention are needed.

First aid and quick transport to a veterinarian with as little stress to the pet as possible are the most important lifesaving steps.

Difficulty Breathing

Upper Airway

The clinical signs of an upper airway problem are different from signs of other types of breathing problems that may have different causes.

The major difference is that upper airway problems involve "noisy" breathing (when a dog or cat is breathing normally, its breathing is usually silent).

- **Noisy breathing happens only if the problem is in the mouth and throat area.**
- **Noisy breathing usually takes place while the pet is inhaling (breathing in).**

The pet's abdomen and chest work much harder to take air into the lungs. The expanding chest rises much higher than normally, and the abdomen looks like it's caving in.

The pet's mouth typically is open while inhaling, and breathing is obviously difficult.

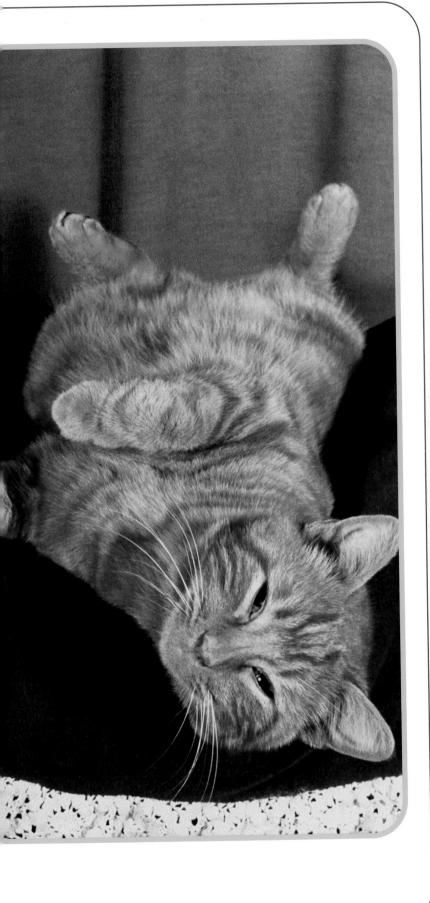

The pet also appears very anxious.

The body temperature can be higher than normal because normally, dogs and cats lose heat while breathing. Dogs and cats do not have sweat glands, so they use their lungs to eliminate body heat. As a result, when their breathing is not normal, their body temperatures can rise quickly. In turn, the breathing difficulty becomes worse when the body temperature rises.

The pet's gum color can be pale white, gray, or blue.

Foreign Objects

A foreign object caught in the throat of a dog or cat is not a common problem, but it happens sometimes with larger dogs. A dog might be playing with an object just big enough to be held easily in the mouth, and that object might become lodged in the throat while the dog is playing and moving. A stick or piece of wood can get caught between the upper or lower teeth, but it usually does not cause a breathing problem.

These animals could die at any moment. The breathing difficulty, or respiratory distress, is immediate and life threatening.

Foreign objects in the throat of cats are very uncommon.

First Aid Recommendations for Foreign Objects

The **Heimlich maneuver** should be performed **when the foreign object can be seen in the back of** the throat. It is usually very easy to see the object.

If the Heimlich maneuver doesn't work, utensils such as cooking tongs can be used to remove the object **when it can be seen.**

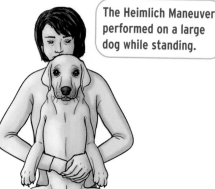

The Heimlich Maneuver performed on a large dog while standing.

Where We Stand

We feel that the Heimlich maneuver should be used only when a first aid provider is certain a foreign object is present and can be seen in the back of the throat. Use of the Heimlich maneuver when there is a breathing problem not caused by a foreign object can harm the animal, especially cats. The Heimlich maneuver can cause injury to the organs of the abdomen. After dislodging a foreign object with the Heimlich maneuver, have the animal examined by a veterinarian as soon as possible.

Do not use your hands and fingers to remove the object. The saliva in the animal's mouth makes the object too slippery, and using your hands will not work. In addition, you may be severely bitten and then be unable to help the animal.

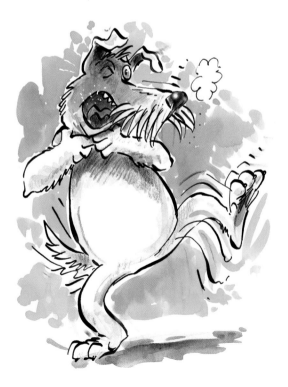

Laryngeal Paralysis

Laryngeal paralysis (which occurs when the larynx becomes paralyzed) is a very common problem in older, large-breed dogs such as Labradors and Golden Retrievers. This happens when the beginning of the windpipe, located in the back of the throat, is unable to open when the dog is inhaling. The different cartilages in the throat stop working and actually close when the dog inhales, blocking air from entering the windpipe. An early sign of this problem can be a change in the pitch or sound of the bark, or the dog may not even be able to bark at all.

Breathing usually becomes very loud and difficult. The loud noise is caused by air being forced in the windpipe through the paralyzed cartilages.

Laryngeal paralysis often is found in pets that have trouble breathing after strenuous or even mild activity. Sometimes the change from cool to warm weather makes laryngeal paralysis more likely to be discovered. Severe difficulty breathing in an obese dog in a warm and humid setting is also typical.

First Aid Recommendations for Laryngeal Paralysis-Related Breathing Problems

Apply cool or cold water over the chest and abdomen.

Keep the dog's stress to a minimum.

Do not put your hands or any utensils in the dog's mouth unless you can see a foreign object while the dog is breathing with the mouth open.

Quick transport to a veterinarian is crucial.

Collapsing Windpipe (Trachea)

Collapsing trachea is a common problem in middle-aged to older small and toy breeds of dogs including the Pomeranian, Poodle, Yorkshire Terrier, and Maltese. The windpipe (trachea) can become weakened and will collapse when the dog is breathing in.

Most dogs with collapsing trachea are obese. The fatty tissue around the mouth and throat worsens the trachea's weakness.

The breathing problems start in a way that is similar to what was described for laryngeal paralysis (above).

A loud, nonproductive, "goose honk" cough happens with a collapsed trachea and usually happens before breathing difficulty starts.

Breathing difficulty usually causes a high body temperature.

First Aid Recommendations for Tracheal Collapse-Related Breathing Problems

Apply cool or cold water over the chest and abdomen.

Keep the dog's stress to a minimum.

Do not put your hands or any utensils in the mouth unless you can see a foreign object while the dog is breathing with the mouth open.

Quick transport to a veterinarian is crucial.

Brachycephalic Syndrome

This syndrome affects dogs with naturally flat faces such as the Bulldog, Pekinese, and Boston Terrier. The syndrome includes smaller-than-normal nostrils, elongated roof of the mouth, smaller-diameter windpipe, and enlarged vocal cords.

Persian and Himalayan cats rarely have difficulty breathing because of the shape of their faces.

Age is not a factor in this syndrome; symptoms can occur in any dog, from young puppies to older adults.

The dog's breathing is usually extremely noisy, and even with an open mouth, it is difficult for the dog to breathe.

The dog usually has a history of "snoring" while asleep or snorting during exercise. Breathing problems can occur during very warm weather. Most owners consider noisy breathing normal for the dog. However, if the dog does not return to normal breathing in a short period of time, the owner should tell the veterinarian.

The dog may have higher-than-normal body temperatures.

First Aid Recommendations for Brachycephalic Syndrome-Related Breathing Problems

Apply cool or cold water over the chest and abdomen if the dog does not breathe normally after a short period of time.

Keep the dog's stress to a minimum.

Do not put your hands or any utensils in the mouth unless you can see a foreign object while the dog is breathing with the mouth open.

Quick transport to a veterinarian is crucial.

Tumors

Tumors in the mouth and throat usually grow slowly and can happen in any breed of dog or cat. They occur mostly in animals that are middle-aged to older. The signs of tumors typically develop slowly over time. Changes in the dog's bark or noisy breathing during mild or heavy exercise may be an early sign. A foul odor in the mouth can also be an early sign of problems.

The pet may have severe breathing trouble.

The pet may also experience noisy breathing and may have higher-than-normal body temperatures.

First Aid Recommendations for Tumor-Related Breathing Problems

Apply cool or cold water over the chest and abdomen.

Keep the dog's stress to a minimum.

Do not put your hands or any utensils in the mouth unless you can see a foreign object while the dog is breathing with the mouth open.

Quick transport to a veterinarian is crucial.

Reverse Sneezing

Reverse sneezes are best described as vigorous and extremely loud snorting sounds that happen rapidly together.

A dog's age and breed have no impact on this breathing problem; it tends to appear suddenly.

When cats have this problem, they will often suddenly begin breathing very rapidly, with their mouths open.

Inhalation may become noticeably difficult.

Early signs in cats may include not wanting to move, or
becoming tired after normal activity.

Cats will cough when they have heart disease or congestive heart failure.

Pericardial Effusion

In older medium to large breeds of dogs, swelling of the
sac that surrounds the heart may occur, resulting in
fluid production (pericardial effusion). When this happens, the fluid build-up can result in heart collapse, and
the heart is no longer able to fill with blood.

Also in older dogs, tumors that develop in the heart can
bleed into the sac that surrounds the heart. The build-
up of blood can also result in heart collapse.

There typically are no early warning signs of pericardial
effusion.

Heart Defects in Puppies and Kittens

Puppies and kittens can have several types of heart defects. Most of these problems are found in puppies and
kittens younger than 6 months of age.

Breeds of dogs that commonly have heart defects include
the Poodle, Maltese, Newfoundland, Boxer, Bulldog, and
Bull Terrier.

Most of the breathing difficulties caused by any kind of
congestive heart failure in dogs and cats happens when
the pet is breathing in.

The mouth usually is open when the pet is breathing in.

Breathing is often very fast, and breaths can be either
shallow or deep. The abdomen usually works hard to
breathe in.

The breathing is not noisy.

Foamy white or red-tinged fluid can come from the mouth
or nose.

Gum color usually is pale or blue.

First Aid Recommendations for Heart Disease-Related Breathing Difficulty

Keep the animal's stress to a minimum at all times! Cats can become very anxious and may bite the first aid provider if too much restraint is used.

Where We Stand

We feel that the single most important step in providing first aid to a cat with breathing problems is to cause the cat as little stress as possible before and during the immediate trip to a veterinarian. There are no home remedies or techniques that will help your cat to breathe.

Wipe any fluid from the nose and mouth area.

First aid providers who can provide oxygen must remember that animals, especially cats, do not like facemasks. Oxygen can be given using the blow-by apparatus placed several inches from the nose and mouth.

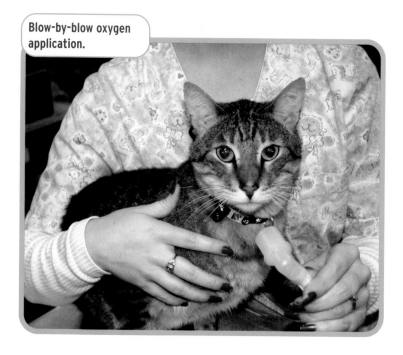

Blow-by-blow oxygen application.

Get the animal to a veterinarian immediately for further treatment.

Lung Disease
Asthma in Cats

Asthma is the number one lung problem in cats. With asthma, the small airway tubes in the lungs are swollen, so air cannot be moved into or out of the lungs.

Any age or breed of cat can have asthma.

Coughing is an early sign of asthma in cats.

Many cat owners believe that cats "cough up" hairballs. Hairballs form in the stomach, and cats vomit hairballs from the stomach. A coughing cat can have the appearance of vomiting. Therefore, the idea that cats "cough up" hairballs probably began because vomiting and coughing look similar.

Cats that cough usually crouch low to the floor or are lying on the floor. The head and neck are stretched out. The mouth is open. The abdomen moves while the cat coughs. Several coughs happen in a row and may end in what appears to be a dry heave (nonproductive vomiting).

Severe asthma can cause breathing difficulty. The cat's breaths are vigorous and labored.

The gums can be pale or blue.

The breathing is not noisy.

There typically is no fluid from the mouth or nose.

Cats may repeatedly roll or turn over on their side when breathing difficulty becomes severe.

Bronchitis in Dogs

Bronchitis (inflammation and swelling of the airways) is a common lung problem in dogs, and it can have many causes. Middle-aged to older dogs are the ones that usually get bronchitis. Dogs with severe dental or gum disease are more likely to develop ongoing bronchitis.

The number one clinical sign before difficulty breathing begins is a continuing and oftentimes severe cough.

Exercise or stress can make the cough worse.

Dogs with bronchitis typically have a dry, hacking cough, which sometimes produces a small amount of sputum (phlegm and saliva). Most dogs will swallow the sputum, and pet owners may not realize it was ever there.

Pneumonia

Aspiration Pneumonia

The most common cause of pneumonia in dogs and cats is called **aspiration pneumonia** and happens when an animal accidentally inhales stomach contents that were produced by vomiting or regurgitation.

Stomach acid and bile are very irritating to the lungs if they are inhaled and may cause severe inflammation.

Aspiration pneumonia can lead to bacterial pneumonia.

Viral and Bacterial Pneumonia

Most cases of viral and/or bacterial pneumonia occur in dogs and cats younger than 1 year of age that were not vaccinated.

This type of pneumonia is highly contagious to other dogs and cats.

Fungal Pneumonia

Fungal organisms in the soil are an uncommon cause of pneumonia in dogs and are a very rare cause in cats.

Digging for gardens or earth-moving for housing developments can release the fungal organisms into the air.

Most dogs with fungal pneumonia show other signs of illness such as weight loss, fevers, and decreased appetite.

Cancer

Tumors in the Chest Cavity

Tumors found in the front part of the chest cavity can produce fluid, resulting in breathing problems in the dog or cat.

Breathing problems tend to develop over weeks.

Most dogs and cats show other signs of illness such as weight loss, fevers, and decreased appetite.

Lung Tumors

Lung tumors are very uncommon in dogs and cats. General signs of illness and coughing are common.

Metastatic Disease

Cancer from other parts of the body can spread (metastasize) to the lungs, resulting in breathing difficulty.

First Aid Recommendations for Lung Disease-Related Breathing Problems

Keep the animal's stress to a minimum at all times! Cats can become very anxious and may bite the first aid provider if too much restraint is used.

First aid providers who can provide oxygen must remember that animals, especially cats, do not like facemasks. Oxygen can be given using the blow-by apparatus placed several inches from the nose and mouth.

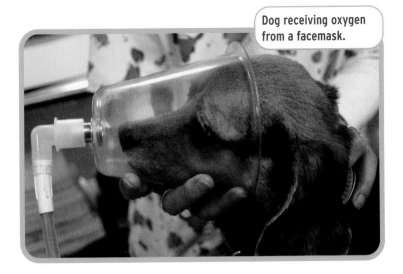

Dog receiving oxygen from a facemask.

Get the animal to a veterinarian immediately for further treatment.

Trauma

Breathing difficulty can often occur as a result of trauma. Please see the complete "Trauma" section for a detailed discussion.

Shock/Collapse

Definition of Shock

Shock is a state of physiological collapse and is accompanied by a weak pulse and other signs.

Shock can occur when not enough blood flows to the body's organs. Poor blood flow that is not fixed could result in failure of the body's organs.

Not enough blood flow to the brain results in collapse.

Shock is always a result of a bigger problem. In order to correctly treat shock, the bigger problem causing the shock must be treated as well.

Clinical Signs of Shock

If you think your pet may be in shock, you must look at the C of the **ABC** concept (assessment of Alertness, Airway, Breathing, and Circulation) and the P of the **RAP** concept (assessment of Respiration, Alertness, and Perfusion, or a blood vessel's ability to inject fluid into a blood vessel to reach an organ or tissue) (see Chapter 3).

The animal in shock may be mentally depressed and may appear unconscious.

The gum color is pale to white.

The **capillary refill time** is very slow or cannot be figured.

The heart rate is higher than normal.

The breathing rate is higher or lower than normal.

Breathing may be difficult.

The pulse is difficult to feel and is faster than normal.

Examples

Animals in shock should be considered triage level 1 victims.

The most common causes of shock include:

- **Any kind of trauma**
- **Any bleeding**
- **Heart failure**
- **Excessive heat (hyperthermia) or excessive cold (hypothermia)**
- **Bloat in dogs**

First Aid Recommendations for Shock

First aid providers should work to get the animal to a veterinarian as quickly as possible.

Slightly lifting the animal's legs can help blood flow to the brain.

Animals that are cold can be wrapped in blankets.

Animals that are hot can have cold water applied to the chest and abdomen.

External bleeding can be controlled.

Trauma

Definition and Mechanisms of Injury

Trauma is simply any physical injury to the body.

Trauma can be either blunt or penetrating.

- **Penetrating trauma means the skin or soft tissue has been broken or penetrated.**
- **Blunt trauma means the skin or soft tissue is not broken or penetrated, but damage may involve internal bleeding.**

Any limb or area of the body can be involved. Blunt trauma can involve multiple areas of the body.

Many injuries caused by trauma are not obvious to the onlooker.

Where We Stand

We feel that a veterinarian should immediately examine any dog or cat that definitely has or even may have suffered trauma.

Common Causes of Trauma in Dogs and Cats

Blunt Trauma

Impact from a Vehicle

Trauma is most commonly caused by an accident in which a dog or cat is hit by any type of vehicle.

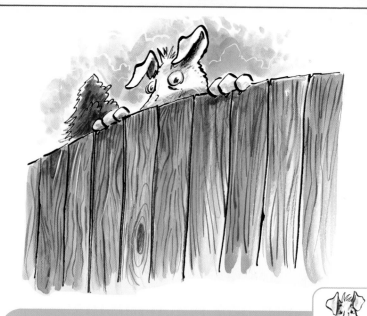

A vehicle can be anything from a scooter to a large truck. Accidents caused by bicycles should also be considered as a possible cause of serious trauma.

Damage to several areas of the body is more likely to happen when the pet is struck by fast-moving and larger vehicles.

Cats and smaller dogs are more likely to be seriously hurt.

Often there is no visible wound after a dog or cat has been hit by a vehicle.

Fall from Any Height

Dogs and cats can be seriously injured when falling from a height as low as 2 to 3 feet.

Most cats and dogs will tend to land feet first, especially cats. Injuries to the limbs and internal organs are common, even when the animal lands on its feet.

Internal injury may not immediately be obvious.

Cats will commonly survive falls from as high as 10 stories, but the internal injuries that may result from the fall are often severe.

When puppies and kittens jump from the owner's lap, serious injuries can result.

Inadvertently Being Stepped On

Puppies and kittens can suffer serious injury if they are accidentally stepped on or fallen on by a child or adult.

Injuries to the limbs are very common after being stepped on.

Caught in Furniture

Reclining chairs and sleeper sofas can easily injure puppies, kittens, small dogs, and cats.

Injuries to the limbs and head are very common.

Caught in Dryer

Some cats like to sleep in secluded areas, including dryers.

Always check the dryer for your cat or kitten before use.

Severe blunt trauma to the head and internal organs as well as heat injury can occur in as little as a few minutes.

Impact from Object

Most pets that are struck by an object are in the wrong place at the wrong time.

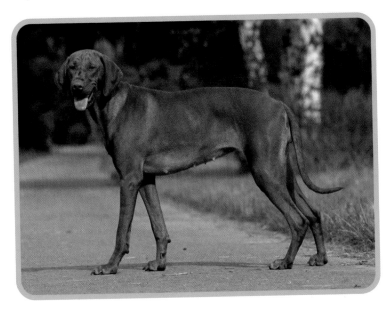

People practicing their golf, baseball, or softball swing should make sure that pets are not nearby, especially kittens and puppies.

Injuries to the head and face are common.

A person's deliberate attack on a dog or cat could result in injury anywhere on the body.

First Aid Recommendations for Any Type of Blunt Trauma

Most, if not all, dogs and cats that suffer blunt trauma are in extreme pain. Even the gentlest family pet can inadvertently seriously bite the first aid provider. Be safe and smart with all injured animals, regardless of the situation.

Proper restraint and transport are the most important parts of first aid to injured animals.

Handle the animal in a way that causes as little stress as possible.

Use muzzles, blankets, and towels to handle the animal.

Try to avoid physically handling an injured animal; instead, place the animal on a board or homemade stretcher.

Secure the animal on the transportation device and get it to a veterinarian immediately.

Do not try to apply **splints** or bandages without proper restraint. This could make the situation worse if the animal becomes more aggressive.

First Aid Recommendations for Broken Bones

Application of Splints

Splints are temporary tools used to stabilize the two or more parts of a broken bone.

Splints can be used in dogs and cats to help prevent further damage to the injured limb.

Splints that are not put on correctly can cause more injury.

Splints should be used only on obvious injuries that are below the knee joint and below the elbow joint.

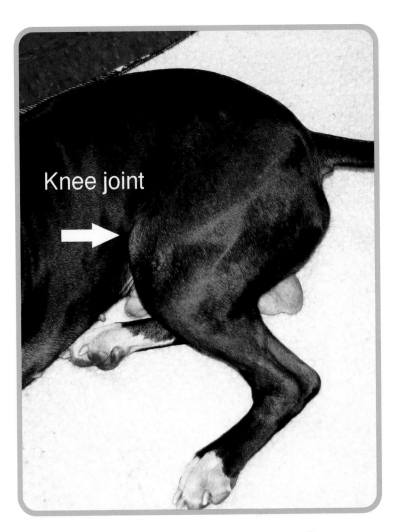

Knee joint

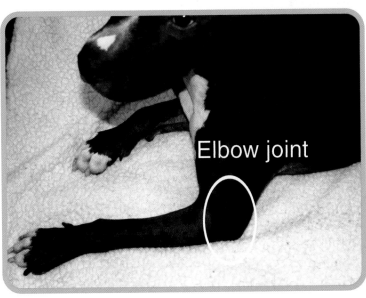

Elbow joint

Splints used on broken bones above the knee and elbow, even if the bone is poking through skin, can cause further injury.

Do not use a splint if you have any doubt about the location of the injury.

Stabilizing the dog or cat on a board or stretcher will also help stabilize the limb.

Any firm material can be used as a splint, from wood to rolled-up newspaper or magazines. Ideally, two pieces of material should be used, one on the inside and one on the outside of the limb.

The splint can be fastened using duct tape, rope, or towels.

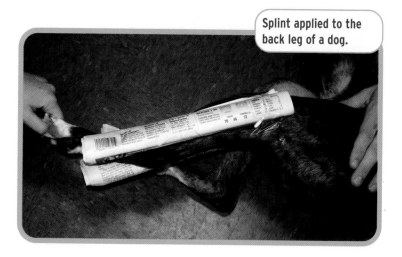

Splint applied to the back leg of a dog.

Alternative to Splints

Wrapping the injured limb that is located below the knee or elbow in thick towels or blankets can work as a splint.

Penetrating Trauma

Gunshot Wounds

Shotgun wounds usually involve a large area of injured tissue and major internal injury, especially if the animal was shot at close range.

Wounds caused by handguns or rifles look like small wounds entering the body. Most wounds related to a single bullet stay inside the animal's body. An exit

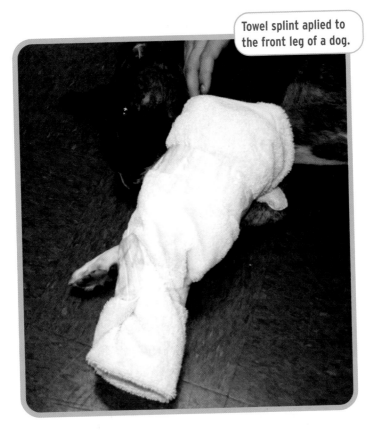

wound can be the same size as the entrance wound or can be larger than the entrance wound. Internal injury is usually massive whether it is to bone, muscle, or internal organs of the limbs, chest, or abdomen.

Linear Objects

Arrows, sticks, and knives are the most common objects that can (and are meant to) penetrate skin.

Injuries can occur anywhere on the body.

First Aid Recommendations for Penetrating Trauma

Proper animal restraint and first aid provider safety are essential before treatment of these wounds.

Gunshot Wounds

Cover bleeding wounds with a towel or blanket. (See "Bleeding" section for details.) There is no need to remove any hair.

Rapid transport to a veterinarian is essential.

Linear Objects

Do not remove the object!

Place towel or bandage around the point where the object entered the limb or body wall.

Do not apply any material if the animal becomes stressed when you try this.

Rapid transport to a veterinarian is crucial.

Blunt and Penetrating Trauma

Fight with Another Animal

Both blunt and penetrating trauma can occur when two animals fight. The risk of both types of trauma increases when one animal is smaller than the other.

Big Dog versus Small Dog

The larger dog typically seizes the small dog in its jaws, gripping the other dog by the neck, chest, or abdomen.

The larger dog then shakes the smaller dog.

The penetrating trauma originates from the actual bite and may appear to be minor.

The blunt trauma affects the tissue and internal injuries when the smaller dog is shaken. Tissue damage beneath the skin can be severe, although no visual sign of such damage may be obvious. The dog in the accompanying photograph had small wounds in the skin but had severe and fatal internal organ damage found during surgery.

Small wounds on a dog with severe internal injury.

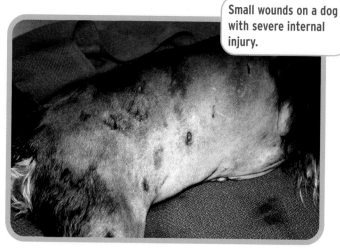

Broken bones and internal organ damage are common.
Any small dog that is attacked by a larger dog needs veterinary attention immediately.

Dog versus Cat

The larger the dog, the more severe the injury to a cat becomes.

Injury to the cat occurs very much as with a small dog attacked by a larger dog (see above).

Cats tend to get very serious internal injuries as a result of being shaken by a dog.

Broken bones and internal organ damage are both common.

Two Dogs of Similar Size

Dogs of about the same size tend to cause superficial wounds like cuts and scrapes.

Bleeding can be either minor or severe. (See "Bleeding" section for details.)

There can be quite a lot of injury to the skin and soft tissues of the limbs and face.

Cat Fights

Wounds received in fights between cats also are usually superficial.

Most cats develop areas of infection (abscesses) days later after the fight.

There are usually no initial injuries, but the abscess can be very obvious.

Infection caused by the abscess could result in a serious illness.

First Aid Recommendations for Blunt and Penetrating Trauma

Most, if not all, dogs and cats that experience blunt and penetrating trauma after a fight with another animal are in extreme pain. Even the gentle family pet can inadvertently bite the first aid provider. Be safe and smart with all injured animals, regardless of the situation.

Handle the animal in a way that causes as little stress as possible.

Use muzzles, blankets, and towels to restrain the animal.

Control bleeding with the use of bandages. (See "Bleeding" section for details.)

Transport the animal to a veterinarian immediately.

Bleeding

Bleeding can be the result of any trauma or injury and can be outside (external) or inside (internal) the body.

External bleeding is obvious and can come from an artery, vein, muscle, or bone.

- **Blood from an artery is bright red in color, and blood flow pulsates.**
- **Blood from a vein is dark red or blue and rapidly oozing, and the flow does not pulsate.**
- **Blood from muscle also is dark red or blue and is slowly oozing, and the flow does not pulsate.**
- **Blood from bone or bone marrow is bright red and oozing, and the flow does not pulsate.**

With internal bleeding, the animal may just appear to be in shock. (See "Shock/Collapse" section for details.)

First Aid Recommendations for Dogs and Cats That Are Bleeding

Proper restraint and use of muzzles are needed before you provide first aid to a bleeding animal.

Wound compression, or direct pressure, is the first and best way to temporarily control bleeding while the animal is taken to a veterinarian. Even if the bleeding comes from an artery, compression should be the first method used to control it. It is better to provide direct pressure to arterial bleeding than to apply a bandage.

A tourniquet should NEVER be applied to control bleeding.

Removal of hair around the wound is not needed.

Application of Bandages

Bandages can be applied to bleeding wounds before transport to a veterinarian.

Bandages are easier to place and fasten on the limbs and the chest or abdomen than on the head of the animal. Any soft, absorbent material can be used as a temporary bandage, including towels, shirts, rags, and diapers. Fasten the bandage with masking tape. Do not use ropes or strings to secure the bandage.

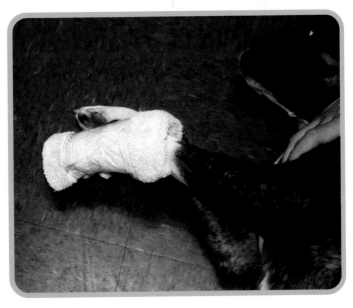

When using tape to fasten bandages to control bleeding of the chest and abdomen, be sure to wrap the tape around the entire animal.

Bandages applied and fastened to the head of the animal must not make breathing difficult. Covering the eyes of the animal could cause stress and excitement, which could result in stronger bleeding or injury to the first aid provider.

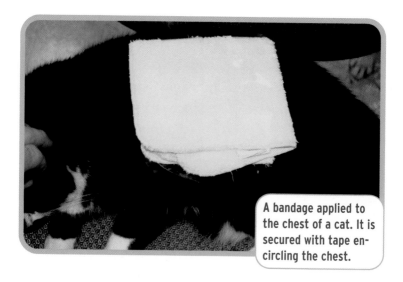

A bandage applied to the chest of a cat. It is secured with tape encircling the chest.

Heat Exhaustion and Heatstroke

Heat exhaustion and **heatstroke** usually occur in the spring, summer, and fall and can occur in any climate.
Dogs frequently suffer from heatstroke.
Cats rarely suffer from heatstroke.
The only way dogs and cats can cool themselves is by panting. Dogs and cats do not sweat like humans. The only true sweat glands in dogs and cats are located on the pads of the feet.
Heavy exercise in moderate climates, especially early in the spring, also can cause problems, even though the outside temperature may not feel very hot.
Obese dogs are more likely to get heatstroke, especially when they are left outside in hot, humid weather, even if the dog is in a shaded area.
In dogs that already have an existing illness like heart disease, heat exhaustion or heatstroke can develop with any amount of activity on a warm day.

Heat Exhaustion

Definition: Heat exhaustion occurs when body temperatures rise to between 103 and 105 degrees F when the animal is active or exercising in warm-to-hot outside (environmental) temperatures.

Heat exhaustion does not cause damage to internal organs.

Heat exhaustion can quickly become heatstroke.

Where We Stand

There is a fine line between heat exhaustion and heatstroke. We feel that all dogs that may have an illness caused by heat should be examined immediately. The difference between life and death could literally be minutes!

Clinical Signs

Excessive panting is typical.

The animal looks for a cooler environment (wood or tile flooring, air conditioning ducts).

Drinking much more water than usual may be a sign.

The animal remains mentally alert (aware and responsive).

First Aid Recommendations for Heat Exhaustion

Apply cold water to the chest and abdomen.

Place the dog in as cool an environment as possible.

Use fans to help cooling.

Provide fresh water.

Heat exhaustion should get better (resolve) within 15 to 20 minutes.

Take the dog to a veterinarian if the animal does not improve or if the animal becomes mentally depressed (unaware and nonresponsive).

Heatstroke

Definition: Heatstroke happens when body temperatures are higher than 105 degrees F and is caused by activity or exercising in warm to hot outside (environmental) temperatures.

Heatstroke is a dangerous, life-threatening condition that requires immediate first aid and veterinary help.

Heatstroke causes damage to internal organs.

Heatstroke can quickly cause death.

Clinical Signs

- **Collapse and shock**
- **Depression or unconsciousness**
- **High heart rate**
- **High and weak pulse rate**
- **Excessive panting or very slow breathing**
- **Bright red or pale white gums**
- **Inability to drink water**

First Aid Recommendations for Heatstroke

Immediately call a veterinarian and notify the staff that you are on your way. The veterinary staff will need to prepare for your dog's arrival in order to provide immediate treatment.

Place the dog in a cool environment. Start your car and place the air conditioner setting on high.

Pour cool water over the entire body, making certain not to get water in the mouth.

Place a fan on the high setting in front of the dog while the car is being cooled.

Place hind legs slightly above the head to help blood flow to the brain and heart.

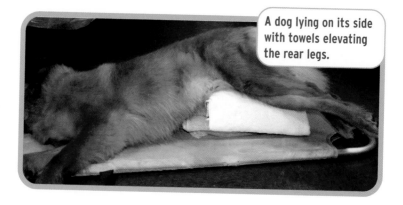

A dog lying on its side with towels elevating the rear legs.

Get the dog immediately to a veterinarian.
Time is critical!

Hypothermia (Body Temperature Lower Than Normal)

Hypothermia can occur in any moderate to cold climate.

Several factors cause hypothermia, including the outdoor or environmental temperature, humidity, wind speed, cloud cover, and ground temperature.

Dogs and cats both suffer from hypothermia equally.

Cats trapped in household refrigerators and freezers have suffered from hypothermia.

Hypothermia can develop even at very moderate temperatures. Even in Hawaii, for example, people can develop hypothermia if they're without shelter on a side of the island where the cliffs and mountains block the sun for most of the day, and during the winter, with wind, rain, waves, and cloud cover.

Definition and Clinical Signs

Hypothermia occurs when the body temperature is lower then normal.

Hypothermia can be mild, moderate, or severe, depending on how ill the animal is and the animal's body temperature.

Mild Hypothermia

Rectal temperatures range between 90 and 99 degrees F.

Signs include mental depression (lack of awareness and response), weakness, and shivering.

Moderate Hypothermia

Rectal temperatures range between 82 and 90 degrees F.

Signs include no shivering, low heart and pulse rate, low respiratory rate, and severe mental depression.

Severe Hypothermia
Rectal temperature is less than 82 degrees F.
Signs include no shivering, coma, no audible heartbeat, difficulty breathing, and dilated pupils.

First Aid Recommendations for Hypothermia
Ensure that the animal is breathing. Perform basic life support (see Chapter 5). You may hear a heartbeat, but it's usually very slow.
Wrap the animal in warm towels.
Place the animal near a source of heat (such as a heating vent).
Take the rectal temperature with a digital thermometer. Most digital thermometers do not register temperatures below 90 degrees F. The reading on the thermometer will be "L" if the temperature is too low to register. The animal should be taken to a veterinarian immediately if the rectal temperature is below 95 degrees F.
Transport the animal inside the vehicle with the heat turned on high.
Actively rubbing the limbs, chest, and abdomen may help.

Abdominal Distention/ Bloat/Torsion

Medium and large breeds of dogs, including the Great Dane, Labrador Retriever, Samoyed, Golden Retriever, Shar Pei, and Bassett Hound, are more likely to have stomach problems.

Definitions and Clinical Signs
Abdominal Distention
Abdominal distention occurs when the stomach area, or abdominal cavity, is enlarged.
The abdominal cavity can increase in size anywhere between the end of the rib cage and the beginning of the hind legs on both sides.

Abdominal distention usually is joined by other clinical signs such as vomiting, pain, shock, or collapse.

Abdominal distention not caused by either bloat or torsion can be caused by internal bleeding, tumors, liver failure, or heart failure.

Bloat

Bloat is a term that simply means the stomach is larger than normal, although it remains in its normal position.

Eating large amounts of food quickly is a common cause of bloat in dogs.

Gas build-up can cause bloat as well.

Abdominal distention, or an increase in abdomen size, is the first sign noticed by pet owners.

The dog may vomit or attempt to vomit.

The gums are typically pink in color, and the heart and pulse rates are normal to slightly fast.

Most dogs are mentally alert.

Bloat is not an emergency requiring surgery, but usually needs veterinary attention to cure the distention.

Bloat must be diagnosed properly. Only an x-ray examination can show whether a dog has bloat or torsion.

Torsion

When a dog's stomach becomes enlarged, it can sometimes twist around on itself. This condition is called **torsion**.

Torsion of the stomach is an emergency that requires immediate treatment.

Only an x-ray examination can show whether a dog has bloat or torsion.

Abdominal distention usually is the first sign noticed by pet owners.

The dog may attempt to vomit, unsuccessfully.

Dogs are very restless and will not lie down.

Torsion of the stomach causes shock and collapse, high heart and pulse rates, pale gums, and depression. Blood flow to the stomach stops during the torsion. Some dogs may have to be carried.

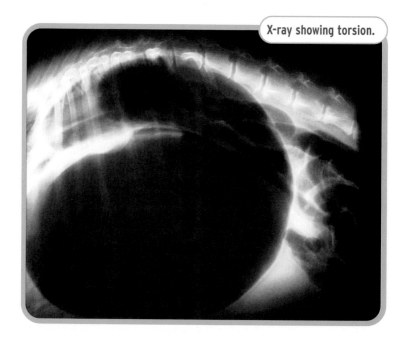

X-ray showing torsion.

The stomach cannot return to the normal position, so immediate surgery is required.

Without surgery, torsion of the stomach will cause death.

First Aid Recommendations for Abdominal Distention

The first aid provider should call a veterinarian immediately after noticing abdominal distention.

The Heimlich maneuver must NOT be used.

Do NOT give any medication such as antacids or anti-gas drugs.

Safely clear any saliva, foam, or vomit from around the mouth and nose.

Do not put pressure on the abdomen.

A board or stretcher may be needed for moving the dog.

Seizures and Fainting

A seizure and a fainting episode can look very similar in dogs and cats.

Seizures usually are caused by disorders of the brain.

Fainting episodes usually are caused by heart or lung problems.

Definition and Clinical Signs

Seizure

A **seizure** occurs when normally steady and rhythmic brain waves are released in an abnormal and jumbled way.

Seizures can occur in both dogs and cats.

The brain waves cause specific physical signs that are different from signs in fainting episodes:

- **Some animals may exhibit more tame behavior or may closely follow the owner before the seizure.**
- **Unconsciousness or lack of awareness during the seizure is typical.**
- **Uncontrollable muscle activity of the entire body may be seen.**
- **Severe shaking may occur.**
- **Leg stiffness may be noted.**
- **The pet's mouth may be closed tightly or wide open.**
- **Urination and defecation are common.**
- **Rectal temperatures usually are higher than normal.**

For some time after the seizure, the animal may seem confused or blind, or occasionally may even act aggressively. This can last from several minutes up to an hour and is not caused by brain damage.

Fainting (Syncope)

Dogs and cats are normal before the fainting episode (syncopal event).

Normal behavior suddenly changes to collapse and unawareness, usually without any shaking of the body, and occasionally with urination or defecation.

Fainting episodes usually last less than 1 minute.

The animal is immediately normal after the fainting episode.

First Aid Recommendations for Seizure

The first aid provider should first contact a veterinarian.

The first aid provider should NEVER reach into the mouth of a dog or cat having a seizure. Dogs and cats cannot "swallow the tongue." The first aid provider may be seriously injured.

Any saliva or foam that builds up during the seizure that makes breathing difficult can be safely wiped away using a large towel or blanket on the sides of the mouth.

The head should be protected from injury during the seizure by using a towel, pillow, or blanket as a pillow.

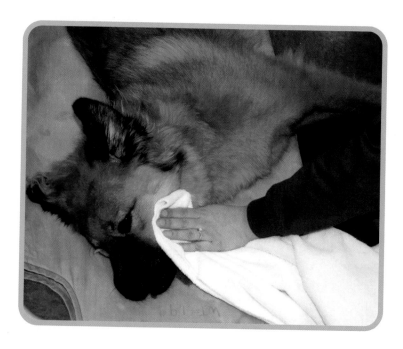

The legs should never be tied together. This can cause serious injury to the animal's bones or joints.

First aid may be needed after the seizure. Make sure that the animal cannot fall down stairs or run into pieces of furniture. Large towels or blankets can be used if the animal behaves aggressively. Use the towels to steady the animal, but do not restrain it. Restraining an animal after a seizure may cause unnecessary excitement or anxiety.

Poisoning or Suspected Poisoning (Exposure to Toxins)

Dogs and cats may eat many items and materials that can be considered poisons, or toxins.

Common drugs that are harmless to people can be very poisonous and even fatal to dogs and cats.

Dogs that chew bottles of medication can be poisoned by the medicine within the bottle.

Many dangerous chemicals can be found within or outside of the household.

Most poisons or toxins eaten by dogs and cats do not have antidotes. Therefore, supportive care by a veterinarian is essential until the animal gets better.

Over-the-Counter Drugs and Medications

Pain Relievers: Nonsteroidal Anti-inflammatory Drugs (NSAIDs)

Aspirin

Aspirin can be used as a pain medication in dogs and cats.

The normal dose for cats is much lower than for dogs.

Aspirin is absorbed rapidly from the stomach into the bloodstream.

Signs of toxicity, or poisoning, include severe vomiting caused by ulcers and kidney failure. Death is possible. There is no antidote for aspirin poisoning (toxicity).

Acetaminophen (e.g., Tylenol)

Acetaminophen is toxic and usually fatal to cats at any dose!

NEVER GIVE ACETAMINOPHEN TO CATS.

Acetaminophen can be given safely to dogs for short periods of time. Giving even appropriate doses for a long period of time can cause toxicity.

Signs of toxicity in cats include difficulty breathing and liver failure, with possible death within 12 hours of eating acetaminophen.

Signs of toxicity in dogs include vomiting caused by liver failure.

An antidote is available for acetaminophen toxicity, but to work it must be given within 1 to 2 hours of eating acetaminophen.

Ibuprofen (e.g., Advil)

Ibuprofen can be used safely in dogs.

Signs of toxicity depend on the amount given. Lower toxic doses can cause stomach ulcers and severe vomiting. Slightly higher toxic doses can cause untreatable kidney failure. The highest toxic dose can cause sudden death.

There is no antidote for ibuprofen toxicity.

Cold Medications

Pseudoephedrine and Phenylephrine (e.g., Sudafed and Neo-Synephrine)

Both ingredients can cause extreme excitement, high blood pressure, muscle tremors, irregular heartbeat, and high body temperatures.

There is no antidote for pseudoephedrine or phenylephrine toxicity.

Pain Relievers

Aspirin, acetaminophen, or ibuprofen may be an ingredient of the cold medication.

Herbal Supplements

Ephedrine-like Ingredients

Herbal supplements for weight loss or stamina contain ephedrine or ingredients that are like ephedrine.

Ephedrine and ephedrine-like ingredients (such as ephedra or ma huang) can cause extreme excitement, muscle tremors, increased body temperature, irregular heartbeat, and possibly death.

There is no antidote for toxicity due to ephedrine-like ingredients.

Prescription Drugs

Pain Relievers

Narcotics (Opioids)

Common pain relievers used for people can contain codeine, oxycodone (Percocet, Percodan, and OxyContin), meperidine (Demerol), hydromorphone

(Dilaudid), fentanyl (Duragesic patches), and hydrocodone (Vicodin).

Narcotics can cause severe depression or unconsciousness in dogs and cats.

Breathing can become severely depressed, and animals may stop breathing.

An effective antidote is available; it must be given through the veins over several hours in dogs and cats that have received toxic doses of narcotics.

Nonsteroidal Anti-inflammatory Drugs (NSAIDs)

Aspirin and acetaminophen are common ingredients in narcotic pain relievers.

Newer anti-inflammatory drugs such as celecoxib (Celebrex) can cause severe stomach or kidney problems in dogs and cats.

Antidepressants

All antidepressant medications can cause excitement, muscle tremors, and high body temperatures in dogs and cats.

There is no antidote for toxicity caused by antidepressants in dogs and cats.

Attention Deficit Hyperactivity Disorder (ADHD) Medications

Most ADHD medications contain amphetamine or amphetamine-like ingredients.

Severe excitement, muscle tremors, and high body temperatures can occur.

There is no antidote for toxicity due to ADHD medications.

Heart Medications

High Blood Pressure Medication

There are safe doses of several kinds of high blood pressure medication for dogs and cats.

Toxic doses can cause shock or collapse, pale gums, and high heart rates.

There is no antidote for toxicity due to high blood pressure medications.

Drugs to Control Irregular Heartbeats (Antiarrhythmic Drugs)

There are safe doses of this kind of medication for dogs and cats.

Toxic doses usually cause very slow heartbeats, shock or collapse, and pale gums.

There is no antidote for toxicity due to antiarrhythmic heart medications.

Environmental Poisonings
Antifreeze (Ethylene Glycol)

Antifreeze commonly leaks on driveways and streets, where dogs and cats lick up the fluid.

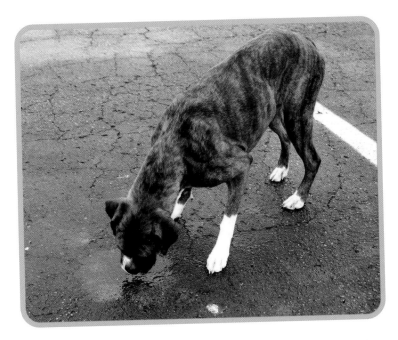

Antifreeze commonly is used to deliberately poison dogs and cats.

Antifreeze is sweet and tastes good to dogs and cats.

The active ingredient, ethylene glycol, is harmless. But the liver changes ethylene glycol to two ingredients that are fatally toxic to the kidneys.

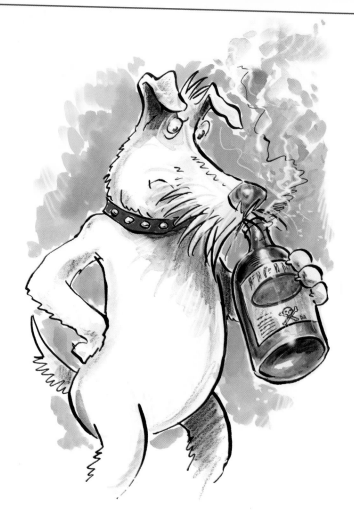

Antifreeze is more toxic to cats than to dogs, as cats go into kidney failure within 8 to 12 hours after eating antifreeze.

Early signs of toxicity in dogs include staggering, vomiting, drinking more water than usual, and urinating more than usual.

Kidney failure takes 24 to 48 hours to develop in dogs.

There is an effective antidote for antifreeze poisoning in dogs and cats.

- **The toxicity must be diagnosed within 4 to 8 hours in dogs and cats for the antidote to work. The antidote keeps the liver from changing ethylene glycol to the two toxic ingredients. Administration of the antidote within 4 to 8 hours can result in a complete recovery, with no effects on the kidneys.**

- Most dogs and cats that get the antidote after 8 hours will die of kidney failure unless they receive a kidney transplant.

Herbicides and Pesticides

Rat and Mouse Bait

These baits contain a very common poison that prevents blood from clotting and causes the animal to bleed to death.

Rat bait and mouse bait taste good and will attract any animal, including dogs and cats.

No signs of poisoning may be noted for 3 to 7 days after eating the bait.

External bleeding may not be noticed unless the animal has an injury such as a cut.

Breathing problems usually are a sign of poisoning caused by internal bleeding in the chest. Shock and collapse also are common signs.

An effective antidote is vitamin K, which can be given along with a blood transfusion even in animals that are in shock. Most dogs recover within 24 to 48 hours once they've been given the antidote and supportive care.

Snail Bait

The active ingredient in snail bait is metaldehyde.

Metaldehyde causes severe shaking, tremors, and seizures that occur within minutes to a half-hour after eating snail bait. Uncontrolled shaking and seizures can cause body temperatures to become extremely high.

Snail bait is considered the tastiest poison to dogs. Dogs will eat every morsel of snail bait available.

There is no antidote for metaldehyde toxicity. Most untreated animals will die of high body temperatures. Supportive care and controlling the seizures are the recommended treatment. Most dogs can recover within 24 to 72 hours with supportive care and seizure control.

Flea, Tick, Ant, and Insect Granules; Vegetable and Fruit Insecticides: Organophosphates

Products found in stores that control ants, fleas, and ticks in your yard can poison dogs and cats.

The same types of ingredients are found in vegetable and fruit insecticides.

Signs occur in one of two phases:

- **Early-phase (seconds to minutes) signs include excessive drooling, diarrhea, vomiting, and urination. An antidote exists for this early phase, and most dogs and cats recover with the antidote.**
- **Later-phase (minutes to hours) signs include excessive shaking, seizures, and paralysis. An antidote exists for this later phase, although it does not always work.**

Mole Bait and Coyote Bait

The ingredient found in mole and coyote bait, although not as easily available, is strychnine.

Strychnine causes uncontrollable seizures and death within a very short period of time after eating it (minutes to hours).

There is no antidote for strychnine poisoning. Supportive care and control of seizures are the recommended treatment. Strychnine can be fatal even with supportive care.

Flea and Tick Products

Most products found in stores that control fleas and ticks on dogs and cats are very safe when used properly.

NEVER apply products labeled for dogs on any cat. Dog products being applied to cats cause the most toxicity.

Clinical signs in cats include severe shaking, seizures, and dilated pupils.

There is no antidote for cats, although supportive care and seizure control will save almost all cats.

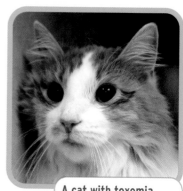

A cat with toxemia.

Spoiled and Moldy Food

Food items that are more likely to grow mold after spoiling include bread products, beans, potatoes, and corn.

Most cases of toxicity occur on or near the day of trash/rubbish pick-up.

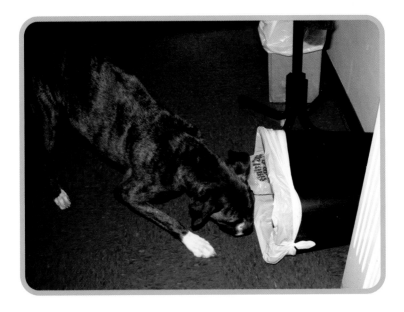

The mold grown on these food items causes shaking, tremors, and seizures in dogs. These symptoms usually follow vomiting.

The ingredient in the mold is quickly absorbed in the stomach (5 to 15 minutes), and shaking or tremors can occur within 30 minutes.

There is no antidote for moldy food. Supportive care and control of seizures are the recommended treatment. Most dogs recover within 24 to 48 hours with supportive care.

Plants: Flowers

Poinsettias

Poinsettias are not toxic to dogs and cats!

The notion that poinsettias were toxic probably came from reports of a very similar-looking, toxic plant. Massive amounts of all parts of the poinsettia plant have been given to dogs and cats without causing death. Vomiting and diarrhea may occur if very large amounts are eaten.

Lilies

Lilies are highly toxic to cats, but not to dogs.

Cats that eat lilies will develop untreatable kidney failure within 12 hours of ingestion.

Where We Stand

Lilies are poisonous to cats and pose more of a threat than any plant, including poinsettias. Please be careful and keep all lilies away from cats, especially indoors during the Easter holiday.

In some cases, the kidney damage may be treatable if the cat is made to vomit up the lily soon after eating it.

There is no antidote for lily toxicity. Once kidney failure happens, most cats do not survive even with aggressive treatment. A kidney transplant may be the only chance to save the cat's life.

Other Plants

Rhododendron

Most rhododendron plants cause irritation to the mouth. Severe vomiting and diarrhea can occur if any plant part is eaten.

There is no antidote. Most animals survive with supportive care.

Azalea

Most azaleas, whether potted indoors or planted outdoors, can cause severe vomiting and diarrhea if eaten.

There is no antidote. Most animals survive with supportive care.

Household Items

Chocolate

Chocolate has several ingredients that can cause toxicity, including caffeine and methylxanthines. The high fat content also may have an effect. Toxicity depends on the type and amount of chocolate eaten:

- **Regular milk chocolate: Approximately 1 ounce per pound of body weight causes toxicity.**
- **Baking chocolate: Approximately $\frac{1}{4}$ ounce per pound of body weight causes toxicity.**

Signs of toxicity start with vomiting and diarrhea. Chocolate can often be seen in the vomit.

The caffeine and methylxanthines then cause severe shaking, tremors, and seizures. Irregular heartbeats also are common.

Death due to seizures and irregular heartbeats can occur within hours after the chocolate is eaten.

There is no antidote for chocolate toxicity. Survival depends strongly on how early the toxicity is discovered and whether supportive care is provided before the start of shaking, tremors, and seizures.

Grapes and Raisins

Recently, kidney failure from eating large amounts of grapes and raisins has been reported in dogs.

The cause is unknown. Clinical signs in most dogs included vomiting.

There is no antidote for grape or raisin toxicity. Supportive care for kidney failure saved 50% of dogs.

Toilet Bowl Cleaner

Commonly used blue toilet bowl cleaner can be very toxic to dogs that like to drink water from the toilet.

The active ingredients include sodium hypochlorite (as in Clorox bleach) and similar chemicals. These ingredients cause chemical burns in the mouth, esophagus, and stomach.

Do NOT make the dog vomit! Chemicals that burn on the way down also will burn on the way up!

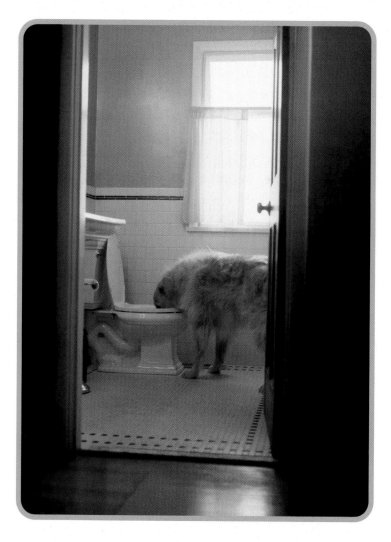

There is no antidote, and supportive care may not save the dog's life.

The best prevention is to avoid use of such products.

First Aid Recommendations for Poisonings

Get the animal immediately to a veterinarian.

Make sure that the animal's airway is clear of saliva or vomit.

The first aid provider should handle excited or overanxious dogs and cats as little as possible. Use towels or blankets to protect your hands and arms from injury.

Pet owners who cause their pet to vomit at home must still get their dog or cat to a veterinarian for further treatment. **Caution:** Vomiting is NOT recommended for some toxins.

Home remedies for poisons or toxins probably will not help the animal.

Early detection or suspicion that the pet ate a toxin is the most important part of successful treatment of poisoning.

Take your pet to a veterinarian if there is the slightest chance that your pet has been exposed to or eaten any potentially toxic substance or medication.

Problems with Urination

In both male and female dogs and cats, kidney or bladder stones can develop that can block urination. Blockage is more common in male dogs and cats.

In dogs and cats that are unable to urinate, life-threatening problems can develop as soon as 24 hours after urinary blockage.

Death can occur after 48 hours of urinary blockage.

Signs

Many dogs and cats may seem like they are repeatedly trying to defecate when the urinary tract is completely blocked.

True constipation is not a common problem in dogs and cats.

Cats will go into and out of the litter box and look as though they are urinating, although they will not urinate. Some cats will be found trying to urinate in unusual places such as sinks and bathtubs and on clothing.

Cats that do not produce any urine within 20 to 30 seconds or that keep trying to urinate may have urinary tract blockage.

Dogs are more likely to look as though they are trying to defecate.

First Aid Recommendations for Urination Problems

First aid providers should be aware that most dogs and cats trying to urinate are probably in a lot of pain in the abdomen. Use care if you must restrain the animal, and handle the animal as little as possible. A muzzle may be needed for some dogs.

NEVER squeeze the bladder or abdomen in hopes of removing the blockage.

Get your pet to a veterinarian immediately.

Inability to Use Limbs

Complete inability to use a limb or limbs is different from limping, or the partial use of the limb.

Complete loss of limb function is an immediate emergency.

First aid usually is needed before transporting the animal to a veterinarian.

One Limb (Front or Back Leg)

Complete loss of function of one limb may be associated with a serious problem.

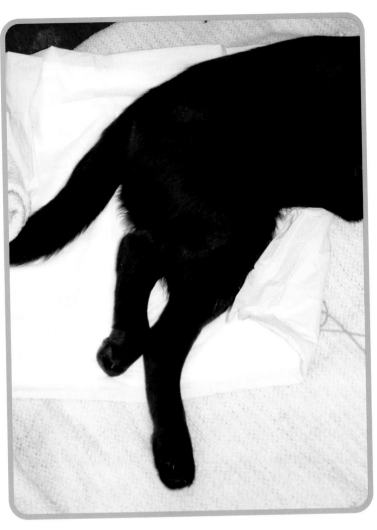

Ligament tears, broken bones, and penetrating injuries are common problems that cause complete loss of limb function.

First Aid Recommendations for Inability to Use One Limb

Dogs and cats may be in extreme pain, requiring the use of muzzles or other kinds of light restraint.

Temporary splints can be applied to injuries below the knee (hind leg) and elbow (front leg); see "Application of Splints" in the "Trauma" section.

Do not attempt to place a splint if the animal will not allow you to restrain it or handle the limb.

Carefully provide transport with as little stress and anxiety to the animal as possible. Use of a board or stretcher may be needed even with injuries to one limb.

Two Limbs

Front Legs

It is uncommon to have an injury to both front legs that causes both limbs to not function.

Trauma can cause both front limbs to be injured.

Puppies that jump from the lap of owners can have injury to both front legs.

Cats that fall from heights can have injury to both front limbs.

First Aid Recommendations for Inability to Use Two Limbs

Animals with injury to both front legs are more likely to not allow restraint and will need muzzles or other ways to protect the first aid provider.

With obvious injuries below the elbow, a temporary splint can be put on each limb.

Dogs and cats that do not allow handling of either limb can have one large splint applied to both limbs. Place a large rolled towel between the two front legs. Place one rolled towel on the side of each limb. Secure the three towels and two limbs.

Secure the animal to a board or stretcher and get to a veterinarian.

Hind Legs

Injury to the spine can cause both hind legs to not function.

Spinal injuries are common when animals are struck by a vehicle.

Signs include complete inability to move either hind leg. The front legs may appear stiff. This is a sign of spinal cord injury.

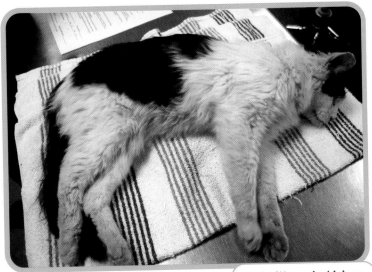

A cat with a spinal injury.

All Four Limbs

Inability to use all four limbs is the sign of a spinal cord injury in the neck.

Trauma is a common cause, although a ruptured disk also can cause inability to use all four limbs.

First Aid Recommendations for Inability to Use All Limbs

Handle the animal as little as possible in order to prevent further spinal injury.

Most dogs and cats will not be able to move the head and may not need a muzzle or a tremendous amount of restraint.

Diabetic Crisis (Low Blood Sugar)

Diabetes is common in dogs and cats.

Occasionally, too much insulin can cause extremely low blood sugar.

Signs of low blood sugar include severe depression, inability to move, collapse, and seizures.

First Aid Recommendations for Diabetic Crisis

Pet owners of dogs or cats with diabetes should have a high-sugar-content syrup on hand at all times.

A small amount of sugar syrup should be placed on the gums of a pet showing any signs of low blood sugar.

First aid providers must be extremely careful not to be bitten when applying sugar syrup to the gums of an animal having a seizure.

Make certain that animals having seizures are not restrained and that the head is protected.

Get the animal to a veterinarian immediately.

Where We Stand

A diabetic crisis is always an immediate emergency. We feel that owners of animals having a diabetic crisis should not wait for sugar syrup to work and should immediately get the pet to a veterinarian.

Difficulty Giving Birth (Dystocia)

Problems giving birth are common in dogs and uncommon in cats.

Difficulties are caused by problems with the mother or problems with the newborn.

Dogs
Problems with the Mother

Earlier injury to the birth canal (pelvis) could make it difficult for normal-size puppies to be delivered. Only an x-ray examination can show if the birth canal is normal. Signs of difficulty caused by injury include severe contractions with no results.

The muscles of the uterus may become tired and may not be able to push the puppies out. Uterus problems can occur in dogs with large litters of puppies or in older dogs. Signs of difficulty caused by uterine muscle weakness may include small contractions with no results or no contractions at all.

Problems with the Puppies

Some puppies can be too large to enter and exit the birth canal. Knowing the father's size can be important. Only an x-ray examination can show whether the puppies are too large.

Certain breeds of dogs may have normal-size puppies, but the shape of the puppy may interfere with giving birth. In Bulldogs, for example, the shoulders of a normal-size puppy may be too wide to pass through the birth canal.

Breech births (in which the puppy is born with hind legs first) account for approximately 50% of all births. Breech is not considered unusual, as it is when a human baby is born.

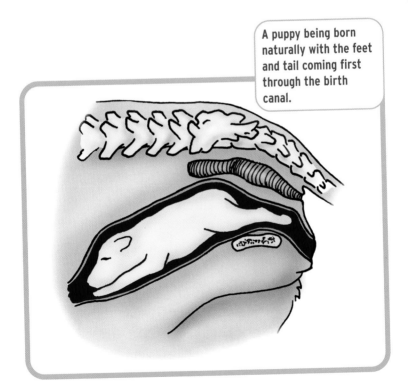

A puppy being born naturally with the feet and tail coming first through the birth canal.

Cats

Regardless of whether the problem is related to the mother or to the kittens, any cat having any difficulty giving birth needs immediate first aid and veterinary help.

When Do You Seek Veterinary Attention?

Cats having difficulty giving birth need immediate veterinary help.

The answer to this question can be very complicated in some dogs.

Many factors are involved, and each mother should be considered on her own.

Knowing the number of puppies to be born can be very important for making decisions. Only an x-ray examination done after approximately 7 weeks after breeding can accurately show the number of puppies.

Several situations require immediate attention:

- **Severe contractions for 15 to 30 minutes with no results**
- **No contractions for 2 hours**
- **Contractions with a bloody discharge that do not produce a puppy**
- **Note: Mothers who seem comfortable even if there have been no contractions for 2 hours may be doing well.**

First Aid Recommendations for Difficulty Giving Birth

Cases in Which Part of the Puppy or Kitten Is Visible

Make certain that the mother is not able to bite you as you handle the puppy or kitten. Muzzles and restraint may be needed.

A sac surrounding the puppy or kitten may or may not be present.

A towel may be needed to grasp the puppy or kitten.

Grab the puppy or kitten by the legs.

Gently pull the puppy or kitten straight DOWN toward the mother's hind legs. Do NOT pull straight backward!

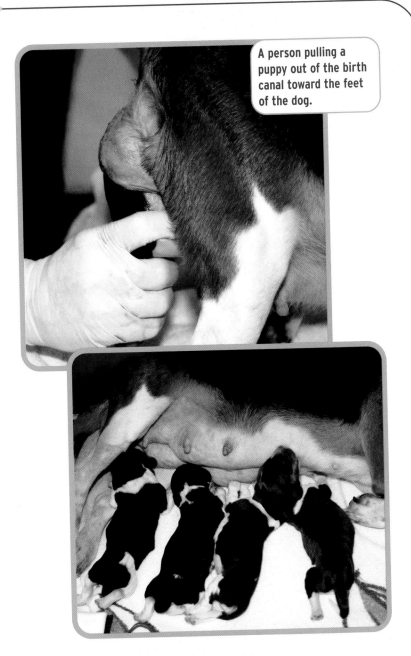

A person pulling a puppy out of the birth canal toward the feet of the dog.

Cases in Which the Puppy or Kitten
May Require Care

Most puppies and kittens have a sac around them when born. The sac should be torn open and removed, starting at the head.

Clear the mouth of all fluid. A suction bulb can help.

Hold the puppy or kitten in both hands with the head pointed toward the ground and vigorously rub the chest to help remove any fluid in the lungs or stomach.

Once the puppy or kitten is breathing and making vocal noises, take care of the umbilical cord as described under "Umbilical Cord Care" (the next list).

The afterbirth may or may not be delivered.

Gently grab the umbilical cord and gently pull down toward the hind legs until the afterbirth is delivered.

Do not panic if the umbilical cord breaks. Use your fingers to clamp over the end of the umbilical cord.

Umbilical Cord Care

Tie the umbilical cord with thread or dental floss approximately ½ inch from the body of the puppy or kitten.

Cut off the afterbirth (if present).

Take care not to pull the umbilical cord too hard.

Once the puppy or kitten is making vocal noise and the umbilical cord is tied, it can be returned to the mother for further care.

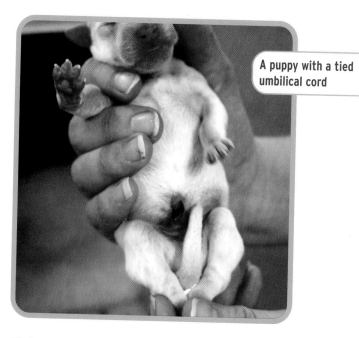

A puppy with a tied umbilical cord

Potential Problems after Giving Birth

Mother

Vaginal Discharge

A small amount of blood or blood-tinged fluid seeping from the vagina is normal immediately after the mother gives birth. There may be a greenish color to the discharge as well.

All discharge should begin to stop after 1 to 3 days.

Vaginal or Uterine Prolapse

Occasionally, part of the reproductive tract can be pushed out of the body after giving birth.

This problem is uncommon but can be life threatening.

A pink or red piece of tissue may be seen hanging from the birth canal.

Do not pull on this tissue.

First Aid Recommendations for Problems in Mother after Delivery

The mother may be showing signs of shock due to internal bleeding.

The mother may be very distressed and may need restraint and a muzzle.

Use gentle direct pressure to stop any bleeding from the tissue.

Get the animal to a veterinarian immediately.

Puppies or Kittens

Breathing Problems

Puppies and kittens may need to have the mouth cleared more than once.

Gently remove any fluid from the mouth or nose.

The gums should be very pink.

Puppies and kittens with breathing problems and pale or blue gums will need immediate veterinary help.

Not Suckling

Puppies and kittens should spend most of their time either suckling or sleeping near the mother.

If the puppy or kitten either is not suckling or is away from the mother, this is a sign of a problem.

Puppies and kittens will become cold quickly.

Place the puppy or kitten in a warm area and call a veterinarian.

Burns

Most burn injuries to dogs and cats are either accidental, but some are deliberate.

Most burn injuries are extremely painful, and the first aid provider should be extremely careful when handling any animal that may be burned.

Hot Water

Hot water can cause moderate to severe burns.

The water temperature lowers quickly after being removed from a heat source.

Water can cover and burn a large area of skin.

The longer the dog or cat's hair, the less likely it is to receive a burn injury to the skin.

Oil or Grease

Oil or grease can produce more severe burns, as it tends to stick to the hair and remains hotter for a longer period of time after being removed from heat.

The first aid provider should be careful not to be burned.

Hot Object

Cats are more likely to jump on a warm or hot stove.

The pads of the feet can be burned. In people, burns on the hands and feet are considered very serious compared with burns to other parts of the body.

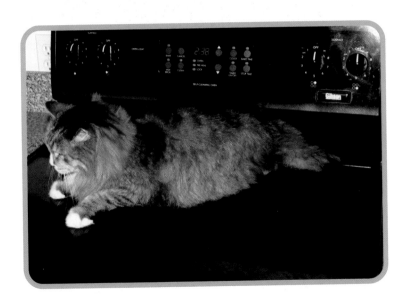

Fire

Unfortunately, all people do not necessarily view dogs and cats in a positive light.

Most unfortunate is the negative feeling some people have toward black cats, especially around Halloween.

Sadly, some people deliberately soak cats with a flammable product (gasoline, lighter fluid) and set them on fire.

The flammable product helps the fire to burn faster and stronger and can cause severe to fatal burns.

First aid is required (see the following recommendations) in most instances. Contact the local authorities as well.

House fires usually cause more smoke inhalation than actual burns. (See "Smoke Inhalation" section.)

First Aid Recommendations for Burns

Be very careful not to become burned by remaining hot oil or grease or to be bitten by the injured dog or cat. Restraint and muzzles may be needed.

Place cool, not cold, water on the area of the burn.

Do not use butter, margarine, or any topical medication on the wound.

First aid providers who own and can use electric grooming clippers can remove the hair over the affected area, especially if oil or grease is the cause of the burn. All of the hair may not be able to be removed, because of pain. Get the animal to a veterinarian immediately.

Snakebites

It is very important to know the kind of snake that bit your pet, in order to treat the pet properly.

Bites from poisonous snakes can result in shock and collapse and possibly death, in addition to severe injury at the wound site.

Nonpoisonous snakebites are nonfatal, yet the bite area can become infected.

Bite wounds usually are on the face or front legs of dogs. (The face is a prime target because of the natural curiosity of dogs.) Snakebite to the limbs usually means that the dog stepped on the snake.

The presence of poisonous snakes depends on where you live. Learn about the poisonous snakes in your area by contacting the local wildlife or park service.

First Aid Recommendations for Snakebite

Snakebites are painful, and the first aid provider should be careful not to be injured. Restraint and muzzles will be needed.

Do not try to kill or capture the snake; you may be bitten as well. A description of the snake's appearance is enough to help the veterinarian treat your pet.

Excessive bleeding can be controlled by direct pressure.

Do NOT place a tourniquet around the limb. The venom will spread despite the use of a tourniquet.

Where We Stand

Removing the venom from the snakebite wound using your mouth does not help and will not decrease the amount of injected venom.

Poisonous versus Nonpoisonous Snakes

Poisonous	Nonpoisonous
Appearance of snake	
Head is triangle shaped.	Head has a thin and straight shape.
The snake generally is shorter with a wider, flatter body.	The snake is thinner and longer in appearance.
Pupils of the eyes are slits.	Pupils of the eyes are round.

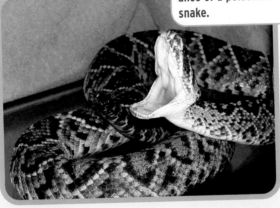

The general appearance of a poisonous snake.

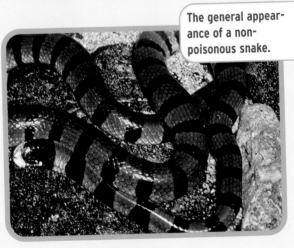

The general appearance of a nonpoisonous snake.

continued

Poisonous	Nonpoisonous
Appearance of bite wound The wound may not be immediately obvious. Usually two distinct puncture wounds are seen with the bite of a poisonous snake. Bleeding and bruising may appear within minutes.	The wound may not be immediately obvious. The wound has the appearance of an upside-down "U." Bleeding may not be immediately obvious. Bruising usually is minimal.

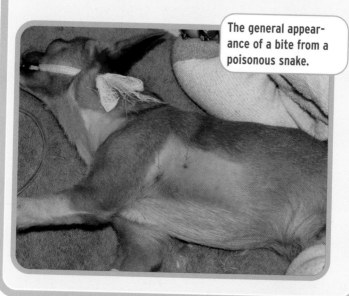

The general appearance of a bite from a poisonous snake.

Signs of shock and collapse may occur. Basic life support CPCR may be needed.

Get the animal to a veterinarian immediately.

Near Drowning

Consequences of near drowning will be different depending on the type of water.

Fresh Water (Lakes, Ponds, Creeks, Rivers)

Fresh water does not build up in the lungs but is rapidly absorbed into the bloodstream.

Many animals will vomit and inhale stomach contents that can harm the lungs.

Lack of oxygen also can damage the lungs.

First Aid Recommendations for Near Drowning in Fresh Water

Do not endanger yourself in an attempt to save an animal from a body of water!

Clear the animal's mouth and nose of any material.

Watch for any attempts to breathe.

Do NOT waste time holding the animal upside down to eliminate water from the lungs.

Basic life support CPCR may be needed if an animal is not breathing.

Animals also can become hypothermic and will require towels or blankets to keep them warm.

Animals that are revived will need to be examined by a veterinarian.

Unresponsive animals should be taken to a veterinarian immediately. Continue to perform basic life support CPCR as long as the animal is not responding.

Salt Water

Salt water is not absorbed well within the lungs. In fact, the salt draws water into lung tissue.

Most of the water in the lungs cannot be physically drained.

Lungs that are filled with water and salt cannot take in and deliver oxygen to the body.

Many animals will vomit and inhale stomach contents that can harm the lungs.

Lack of oxygen also can damage the lungs.

First Aid Recommendations for Near Drowning in Salt Water

Do not endanger yourself in an attempt to save an animal from the ocean, especially in the case of high waves and rip tides.

Immediately raise the animal up so that the rear half of the body is higher than the front half.

Perform 3 to 4 quick chest compressions to remove any obvious water from the lungs or windpipe.

Clear the airway of any material.

Watch for any attempts to breathe.

Basic life support CPCR may be needed in animals that are not breathing.

Immediate transport to a veterinarian is recommended. Continue to perform basic life support CPCR as long as the animal is not responding.

Swimming Pool Water

Near drowning in a swimming pool is similar to that in fresh water.

Chlorine can be irritating to the lungs, in addition to the other problems associated with near drowning in fresh water.

First Aid Recommendations for Near Drowning in Swimming Pool

Follow the same recommendations as those for near drowning in fresh water.

Smoke Inhalation

Fire

Smoke can physically damage the lungs, making it difficult to breathe and making it difficult for the lungs to provide oxygen to the body.

Smoke also can contain the invisible gas carbon monoxide.

Carbon monoxide prevents normal red blood cells from carrying oxygen.

The combination of physical damage by smoke and carbon monoxide can make treatment very difficult.

Trapped in Garage with Running Car

Carbon monoxide is an invisible gas with no smell that is released from car exhaust.

Toxic levels of carbon monoxide can build up with running cars in a garage with the garage door raised only a small amount.

Where We Stand

Pet owners may warm up the car in the garage during the winter time with the garage door raised only a small amount. We feel that the garage door should be raised completely to prevent toxic levels of carbon monoxide from building up.

First Aid Recommendations for Smoke Inhalation

First aid providers at the scene of a fire should follow instructions given by fire department personnel.

Do not enter a burning house!

Getting yourself injured could prevent you from helping a family pet.

Pets should be moved as far away from smoke as possible.

Follow the ABCs of resuscitation, and make sure that the airway is clear of any material and that the animal is breathing.

Basic life support CPCR may be needed.

If available, oxygen can be given to the animal, by facemask or blow-by apparatus.

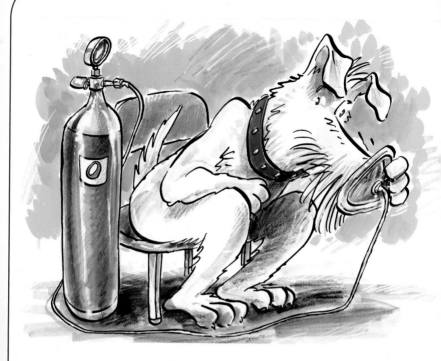

Giving oxygen is the main treatment for carbon monoxide poisoning. Oxygen speeds carbon monoxide out of the body.

Get the animal to a veterinarian, giving oxygen at all times.

Allergic Reactions

Anaphylactic Reactions

True **anaphylaxis** usually occurs as a result of vaccinations, while the pet is still at the veterinary office. The reaction comes on extremely quickly.

Signs include collapse, shock, white gums, high heart rate, weak pulse, and breathing difficulty

Occasionally, bee stings can cause the same type of reaction, with the same signs.

First Aid Recommendations for Anaphylactic Reactions

Keep the airway clear.

Raise the hind legs so that they are higher than the head.

Perform basic life support CPCR if breathing stops.

Wrap the animal in a towel or blanket to keep it warm and get it to a veterinarian immediately.

Do not attempt to give any medications.

Facial Swelling and Hives

Allergic reactions caused by bee or wasp stings are very common in dogs and uncommon in cats.

Dogs have many cells in the skin that respond to an allergic reaction by releasing a substance called histamine.

Histamine causes swelling, bright red color of the skin, and small skin bumps called **hives**.

This type of allergic reaction can become true anaphylaxis with shock and collapse, but this is not common.

First Aid Recommendations for Hives

Giving an antihistamine by mouth will probably not stop the allergic reaction in most affected dogs.

Many dogs will seem irritated and may scratch excessively.

Where We Stand

Pet owners and first aid providers should never place any drops or ointment in the eye of a dog or cat before the animal is examined by a veterinarian. Some eye drops and medications can be harmful if given for the wrong eye condition

Make certain that the dog has a normal airway and is breathing normally, and get it to a veterinarian, where injections can be given to stop the reaction.

Eye Problems

Any and all problems with the eyes in dogs and cats are considered a medical emergency, and require immediate examination by a veterinarian. Any unnecessary delay could result in permanent damage to the eye and loss of sight.

"Red Eye"

The tissues surrounding the eye include the sclera (white portion of the eyeball) and the conjunctiva (lining of the eye socket beneath the eyelids).

Irritation to either of these areas can cause the eye to look red.

Blood can appear within the eyeball and make it look dark red.

Causes of red eye include glaucoma (increased pressure within the eyeball), conjunctivitis (inflammation of the lining of the eye socket), or infection around or within the eye.

Excessive Blinking

Irritation of any parts of the eye can cause excessive blinking.

Scratches on the cornea (clear surface of the eye), infection within or around the eye, and glaucoma can cause excessive blinking.

Excessive blinking is a sign of pain within or around the eye.

Closed Eye

Severe damage or eye infection can cause the animal to close its eyelids.

Do not attempt to open the eyelids!

Eye drainage (discharge)

- **Any eye problem can result in drainage or discharge from the eye.**
- **The discharge can be clear, green, white, light brown, red, or any combination.**

Do not provide any first aid beyond gently removing any discharge from beneath or around the eye.

Immediate veterinary help is needed.

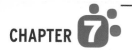
FIRST AID FOR TRIAGE LEVEL 2 PATIENTS

Definition

Triage level 2 patients usually survive if they receive simple care within a few hours.

First aid and transport to a veterinarian are important to diagnose the problem and treat it properly.

Giving medication at home without a veterinarian's recommendation and waiting for long periods of time to seek veterinary help can be dangerous!

Where We Stand

We discourage home treatments without a veterinary recommendation for triage level 2 patients. We especially discourage giving any over-the-counter medication to dogs or cats that are vomiting or have diarrhea. You can often prevent a triage level 2 problem from worsening to a triage level 1 problem with an examination by your veterinarian, whether on an emergency basis or by appointment. Let's say that your dog has been vomiting for several hours, and now the vomit contains blood. Whatever the cause of the vomiting, your pet can rapidly become severely dehydrated, and the vomiting's cause could be very serious. Giving the dog Pepto-Bismol or Kaopectate and then waiting could be very harmful. Continued vomiting, especially if the vomit contains blood, requires examination by a veterinarian.

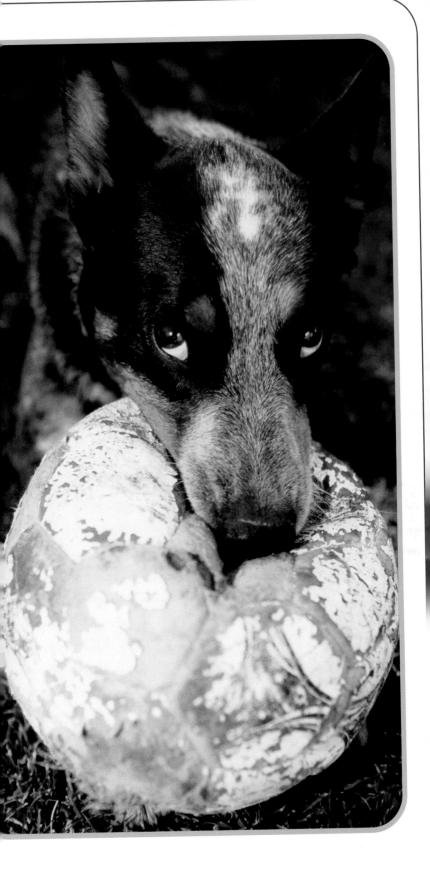

Vomiting and Regurgitation

Definitions

Vomiting

Vomiting is an active process that originates from the stomach or intestines.

Regurgitation

Regurgitation is a passive process that begins at the esophagus (which runs from the throat to the stomach)

Clinical Signs

Vomiting

Dramatic, even violent movement of the abdomen occurs. The brain sends signals to the stomach to get rid of its contents. Therefore, the stomach must be involved to cause vomiting.

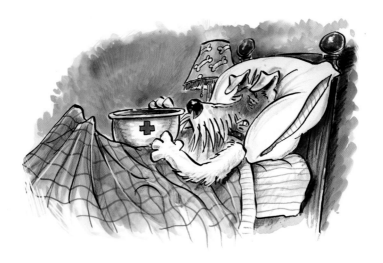

Salivation (drooling) may be noted before the animal vomits.

The mouth is usually open.

Vomit is hurled out of the mouth.

Vomited material can consist of partially digested food, clear fluid, white foam, yellow or green fluid (bile), reddish brown fluid (that looks like coffee grounds), blood and blood clots, or a combination.

Regurgitation

The abdomen does not move. No signal to the brain occurs that tells the stomach to get rid of its contents, because the problem occurs *before* the stomach. No signal is sent to the brain to activate the esophagus either. The esophagus acts on its own—it does not depend on signals from the brain.

The dog or cat may appear to start coughing or choking as regurgitated material enters the throat and mouth.

Some dogs and cats may have trouble breathing as a result of inhaling material (aspiration pneumonia). This may be the only sign of regurgitation.

Regurgitated material is either fresh food with white foam (not digested) or just clear or white foam. The material should be colorless because all fluid originates before the stomach or intestines.

Causes

Vomiting

There are over 75 different causes of vomiting in dogs and cats! Many of the causes have very different treatments and are discovered with a specific type of test.

Regurgitation

Problems with the esophagus cause regurgitation.

Foreign objects can cause the esophagus to be blocked.

The esophagus can stop working and not move food and water to the stomach. The food and water build up until the animal regurgitates

First Aid Recommendations for Vomiting and Regurgitation

Ongoing vomiting may be a sign of a serious problem and requires veterinary help.

Regurgitation is always a sign that veterinary help is needed.

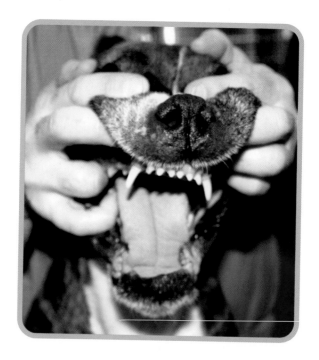

Keep the airway clear, and be careful not to place your hands or fingers within the animal's mouth.
Do not use the Heimlich maneuver!

Diarrhea

Diarrhea can come from the small intestine, the large intestine, or both. The origin of the diarrhea is important, as it can help you or the veterinarian to figure out its cause and treatment and how well the animal will recover.

Small Intestinal Diarrhea

Clinical Signs

- Normal to slightly more defecations per day
- Large amounts of diarrhea
- Brown in color with no mucus or blood
- Black diarrhea seen in some cases

Causes

There are over 75 different causes of diarrhea in the dog and cat!

122

Black diarrhea is a sign that there is bleeding within the intestines.

First Aid Recommendations for Small Intestinal Diarrhea

Black diarrhea combined with pale gums and depressed or lethargic behavior should be considered a triage level 1 situation. The animal needs to be taken immediately to a veterinarian.

Do not give any medication without a veterinarian's recommendation.

Dogs or cats in pain could accidentally harm the first aid provider.

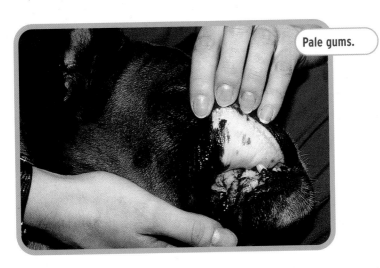

Pale gums.

Large Intestinal Diarrhea (Colitis)

Clinical Signs

- More frequent defecations
- Straining (pushing hard with no results) to defecate
- Small amounts of feces
- Feces may contain mucus or fresh blood.

Potential Causes

Colitis can be caused by parasites (whipworms in dogs), eating something harmful or inappropriate, polyps in the colon, food allergy, or immune problems.

First Aid Recommendations for Large Intestinal Diarrhea

Do not use the Heimlich maneuver in a dog or cat straining to defecate.

Do not remove any material that may be coming from the anus.

The presence of blood means that the animal needs to be taken to a veterinarian.

Combined Vomiting and Diarrhea

Vomiting and diarrhea happening at the same time can be from any of the causes listed for each condition and may be a sign of a more serious problem than when vomiting and diarrhea occur separately.

Ongoing vomiting and diarrhea can cause the animal to lose large amounts of fluid and become dehydrated, regardless of the cause.

First Aid Recommendations for Combined Vomiting and Diarrhea

Do not give a dog or cat medication without a veterinarian's recommendation.

Keep the airway clear and take the animal to a veterinarian.

Lacerations (without Excessive Bleeding)

Lacerations (cuts) do not always bleed a great deal.

Minor dog bites, cat fights, contact with fences and other sharp objects, and scissors accidents are all common causes of lacerations.

Some pet owners may be tempted to use home remedies.

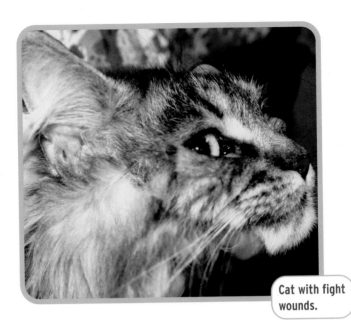

Cat with fight wounds.

First Aid Recommendations for Lacerations

Use grooming clippers to remove the hair from around the laceration.

Do not apply any topical medication (creams, ointments) to the laceration.

Most lacerations will need to be sewn (sutured) by a veterinarian.

The sooner the laceration can be treated, the faster the healing can begin.

A bandage can be put on the wound to keep it clean and protect it from germs. (See "Bandaging" in Chapter 6: First Aid for Triage Level 1 Patients.)

Nosebleeds

Bleeding from the nose can come from one or both nostrils of dogs and cats.

Excessive sneezing can occur.

Possible causes include infection, bleeding disorders (including bleeding problems from rat poison), nose tumors, foreign objects, immune disease, and trauma.

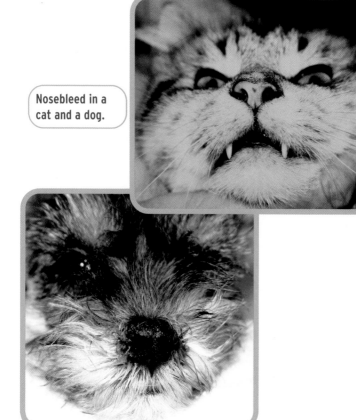

Nosebleed in a cat and a dog.

A continuing nosebleed combined with depressed or lethargic behavior and pale gums is a triage level 1 situation, and the animal needs to be taken immediately to a veterinarian.

First Aid Recommendations for Nosebleeds

Do not place anything in the nostrils!

Be very careful not to make breathing difficult when applying gentle compression to the nostrils with a towel.

Take the animal immediately to a veterinarian.

Blood in Urine

Blood can appear in the urine of a male or female dog or cat with or without straining to urinate (trying to urinate, with no results).

Possible causes include infection, bleeding disorders (including bleeding problems from rat poison), bladder tumors, and trauma.

Blood in the urine combined with depressed or lethargic behavior and pale gums is a triage level 1 situation. Get the animal immediately to a veterinarian.

Blood in the urine of a dog or cat that is straining to urinate is a triage level 1 situation. Get the animal immediately to a veterinarian.

Blood can be in the form of clots or mixed with the urine.

First Aid Recommendations for Blood in Urine

Do not place anything in the vulva or penis!

Gentle compression can be applied with a towel over the vulva or penis if blood is dripping or flowing.

Get the animal immediately to a veterinarian.

Blood in Bowel Movement

Blood in a bowel movement, combined with depression or lethargic behavior and pale gums, is a triage level 1 situation.

Blood in the feces can happen with or without diarrhea.

Blood suggests that the large intestine is involved.

Blood can be bright red, with or without blood clots.

The blood can appear within diarrhea as slimy and mucus-like.

The dog or cat may be straining to defecate.

First Aid Recommendations for Blood in Bowel Movement

Do not place anything in the anus!

Gentle compression can be applied with a towel over the anus if blood is dripping or flowing.

Get the animal immediately to a veterinarian.

Rectal Prolapse

The inside part of the large intestine (rectum) can begin exiting the anus in dogs and cats that are straining to defecate or urinate; this condition is called **prolapse** (See "Straining to Urinate" in Chapter 6; First Aid for Triage Level 1 Patients.)

Female dogs and cats having problems giving birth can strain enough to cause prolapse of the rectum.

Puppies and kittens with a lot of worms and also diarrhea are most likely to have this problem.

A prolapse of the rectum will look like a small tubular piece of pink tissue coming from the anus.

First Aid Recommendations for Rectal Prolapse

A prolapsed rectum can be painful, and the first aid provider should be very careful not to be bitten.

Do not try to push the rectum back into the anus!

Do not put any topical medication on the anus.

Cover the tissue coming out of the anus with a warm, moist towel, and transport the pet to a veterinary facility.

Loss of Balance

Cats and older dogs can have a disorder of the **vestibular nerve**. This nerve is linked to the ear and helps animals keep their normal balance.

The cause of vestibular disease is not known.

Cats and older dogs may vomit once or twice, may tilt the head to one side, may have problems standing up, may fall to the same side or may fall down a lot, and may have trouble staying on one side only.

The eyes move rapidly back and forth.

Animals may feel as if they have been spun around extremely fast.

Inner ear infections can cause the exact same signs but may occur in a dog or cat of any age.

The ears usually have an odor or discharge, and the animal may shake its head excessively. (See "Ear Problems" in Chapter 8: First Aid for Triage Level 3 Patients.)

First Aid Recommendations for Loss of Balance

Dogs or cats with vestibular or inner ear problems may be very anxious. The first aid provider should be careful not to be injured.

Restrain these animals as little as possible using large towels or blankets.

The signs are similar to signs of motion sickness in people, although there is no medication known to help these animals.

Some animals may require veterinary help and support.

Problems Associated with Breeding in Dogs

Male: Penile Problems

The outer covering of the penis is called the **prepuce.**

The penis can remain extruded, or sticking out, from the prepuce after breeding or attempts at breeding.

The prepuce can keep blood from moving out of the penis and prevent blood flow.

The result is an engorged penis, with tissue that can die due to lack of blood flow. The medical term is **paraphimosis**. Paraphimosis can kill the dog.

The urine leaves the body from the penis through the urethra as well.

An engorged penis not only is extremely painful but can keep the dog from urinating normally and cause a blockage. (See "Difficult Urination" in Chapter 6: First Aid in Triage Level 1 Patients.)

First Aid Recommendations for Penile Problems

Paraphimosis is extremely painful.

The first aid provider should be extremely cautious when handling dogs for transport.

Muzzles and restraint may be needed.

There are no home remedies that can help.

The dog needs to be brought to the veterinarian as soon as possible. Paraphimosis is extremely treatable when found and treated early.

Female: Blood from Vulva Due to Traumatic Mating

Trauma to the female dog happens sometimes during mating.

In the normal act of mating between a male and a female dog, the male dog is "locked" with the female for a period of time. Intercourse has happened, but the penis must decrease in size before exiting the vagina. The period of time is not predictable.

The male and the female dog should be allowed to get into a comfortable position during the locking period.

Dogs that struggle during this time could cause trauma to the female dog.

Blood can come from the vulva if trauma has taken place.

First Aid Recommendations for Blood from Vulva

Be careful not to be bitten by either dog during the locking period.

Use gentle compression of the vulva with a towel.

Do not place anything in the vulva! Bleeding from traumatic mating is not the same as the menstrual cycle.

Get the animal to a veterinarian.

CHAPTER 8

First Aid for Triage Level 3 Patients

Definition

- Triage level 3 patients have minor injuries or illnesses that can wait for treatment while other, more critically ill or injured patients receive needed care.
- First aid can be used, although veterinary help is needed to properly diagnose and treat the problem.
- Giving medication at home without a veterinarian's recommendation can be dangerous!

Where We Stand

Home treatment without a veterinarian's advice is not recommended with triage level 3 minor injuries. We especially discourage giving any over-the-counter medication. Examination by your veterinarian can keep a triage level 3 problem from worsening to a triage level 1 or 2 problem.

For example, your cat may be lethargic and have runny eyes and a runny nose. People may take cold medicine that contains acetaminophen (Tylenol) for similar symptoms. But giving acetaminophen to your cat can be fatal, because acetaminophen is extremely toxic to cats.

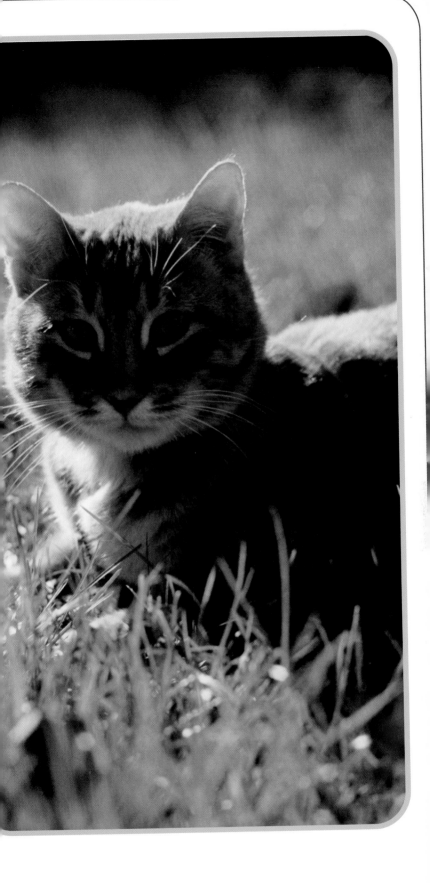

Sneezing

Dogs

Productive

With productive sneezing, material actually appears from the nostrils. The color and consistency of the material produced can help to identify the cause of the problem:

Clear, thin liquid

- Most dogs that occasionally sneeze clear liquid can be considered normal.
- Constant sneezing of clear fluid could indicate a foreign object in the nose such as a blade of grass or seed awn (or burr).

Thicker material (often noticeably discolored)

- Material may be light brown, brown, or greenish in color.
- Any infection of a nostril could cause the production of material that is thick and has some color.
- Ongoing infections or even tumors in the nose could result in the production of thick material from the nose after sneezing.

Blood or blood-tinged fluid (see Chapter 7: First Aid for Triage Level 2 Patients)

- Production of blood could mean a very serious problem such as a bleeding disorder, tumor, or severe infection.
- Examination by a veterinarian is needed soon.

Nonproductive

General irritation of the nose can cause sneezing.

There typically is no material produced with the sneeze.

Causes could include breathing in an aerosol, dust, dirt, and any other small particle.

This kind of sneeze does not usually cause continuous sneezing.

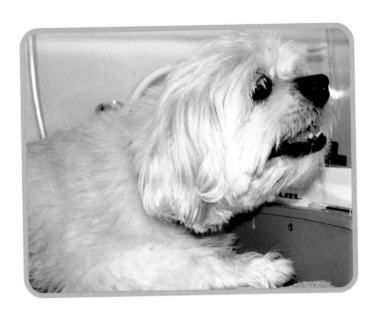

First Aid Recommendations for Sneezing in Dogs

Clear the dog's nostrils of any fluid or any dried material. A dog breathing with the mouth open usually has nostrils that are completely filled with material and could be classified as triage level 1. This animal needs immediate help.

Cats

Productive

The color and thickness of the material produced can help you or the veterinarian to figure out the cause of the problem.

Clear, thin liquid

- Most cats that occasionally sneeze clear liquid can be considered normal.
- Constant sneezing with clear fluid could mean there is a viral infection or a foreign object in the nose such as a blade of grass, a seed awn, or a benign (non-cancerous) mass called a polyp.

Thicker material (often noticeably discolored)

- Material may be light brown, brown, yellow, or green-ish in color.
- Any infection of a nostril could cause the production of material that is thick and has some color.
- Ongoing infections could result in the production of thick material from the nose after sneezing.
- Tumors of the nose are uncommon in cats.

Blood or blood-tinged fluid (see Chapter 7: First Aid for Triage Level 2 Patients)

- Production of blood could mean a very serious problem such as a bleeding disorder or severe infection.
- Examination by a veterinarian is needed soon.

Nonproductive

General irritation of the nose can cause sneezing.

There typically is no production of material.

Causes could include breathing in an aerosol, dust, dirt, and any other small particle.

Occasionally, benign tumors called polyps can cause nonproductive sneezing.

This kind of sneeze does not usually cause continuous sneezing.

First Aid Recommendations for Sneezing in Cats

Clear the nostrils of any fluid or any dried material. Be careful not to get bitten.

A cat breathing with the mouth open usually has nostrils that are completely filled with material and could be classified as triage level 1. This animal needs immediate help.

Polyps in a cat caused by sneezing.

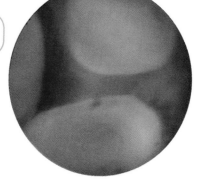

Reverse Sneezing in Dogs

A reverse sneeze can be a very dramatic event!

Description

Many dogs can appear to be having severe breathing difficulties.

The difference between a reverse sneeze and a regular sneeze is that with reverse sneezing, the efforts are inward rather than outward.

The reverse sneeze is a noisy, snorting sound that repeats several times.

Some dogs can have a bluish tongue.

The sneezing starts and stops abruptly.

Dogs are normal before and after the reverse sneeze.

No fluid is produced from the nose.

Reverse sneezing is uncommon in cats.

Cause

The cause of a reverse sneeze is irritation of the back of the throat or nose.

Dogs with allergies can develop a reverse sneeze.

A foreign object such as a blade of grass or other plant material can cause a reverse sneeze.

First Aid Recommendations

A reverse sneeze is not a sign of breathing difficulty.

However, the reverse sneeze may be difficult to tell from a breathing difficulty.

Call your veterinarian or veterinary emergency facility if you have any doubts!

Coughing (with No Difficulty Breathing)

Dogs
Productive

Bronchitis

- Inflammation of the airways (bronchi) from any reason can cause a moist, productive cough.
- Material produced in coughing can be white (normal mucus), brownish white (from infection), or blood tinged.
- Dogs frequently swallow material produced during and after coughing.
- Most dogs with bronchitis also show general signs of being ill, including lack of appetite, decreased activity, and general sluggishness.

Heart Disease

- Fluid in the lungs that builds up as a result of congestive heart failure can produce a moist, productive cough.
- Material produced in coughing can be clear or blood tinged.
- Most dogs that cough because of congestive heart failure have breathing difficulty.

Heartworm Disease

- One of the first signs of heartworms is a moist, productive cough.
- The heartworms live in the part of the heart that delivers blood to the lungs.
- A cough is the first sign of problems. It occurs well before any signs of heart failure.

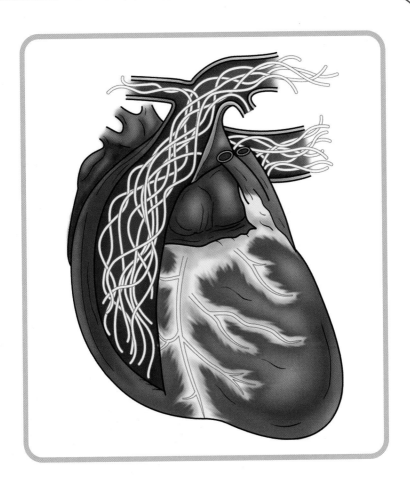

Pneumonia

- Any cause of pneumonia produces a moist cough that usually produces mucus or infected material.
- Most dogs become very ill with fever and are not eating or drinking.
- "Walking pneumonia" is a term used in human medicine that describes a person with pneumonia who is still able to function and does not need to be hospitalized. Most dogs with pneumonia are very ill, however, and will need to be hospitalized even if they do not have difficulty breathing.

Nonproductive

Kennel Cough

- Kennel cough is an infectious disease that dogs catch very easily.
- Dogs vaccinated for kennel cough can still get kennel cough, although the strength and length of illness are much less than in unvaccinated dogs.
- The cough is dry and continuous and can happen with mild exercise or even the normal pressure from a collar.
- Dogs may seem to swallow material after the coughing episode, but this type of cough is not usually productive.

Collapsing Trachea

- Small breeds of dogs can develop weakness in the windpipe (trachea).
- A cough usually develops well before respiratory distress. (See "Difficulty Breathing" in Chapter 6: First Aid for Triage Level 1 Patients.)
- The cough is a "goose honk" type of sound and is dry (nonproductive).
- The cough can happen with mild exercise or even the normal pressure from a collar.
- Dogs may seem to swallow material after the coughing episode, but this type of cough is not usually productive.

Heart Disease

- An enlarged heart can push on the windpipe and cause a nonproductive cough well before signs of breathing difficulty appear.
- Dogs can appear normal, just as with kennel cough and collapsing trachea.

Cats

A veterinarian should examine a cat that coughs even if the cat is not having difficulty breathing.

Coughing and vomiting may look similar in cats.

Cats do not "cough up" hairballs!

Cats *vomit* hairballs.

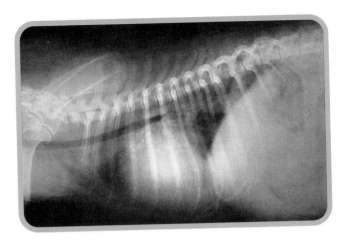

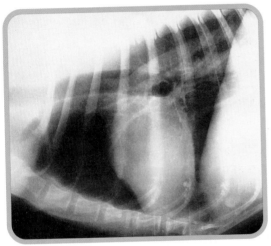

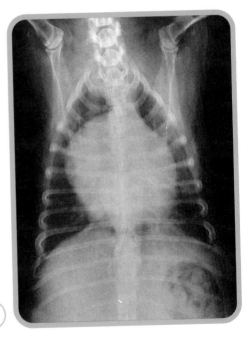

Enlarged heart in a dog.

141

Where We Stand

Cats do not "cough up" hairballs. This expression likely comes from the fact that the acts of vomiting and coughing appear similar in cats. Occasionally, cats will begin to "hack" before vomiting. However, a "hack" can actually be a cough. Coughing is never normal in cats. Please have a veterinarian examine your cat if you feel that it may be coughing. Veterinarians often see cats in advanced stages of asthma for the first time because the pet owners thought that the coughing and breathing problems were from "coughing up" hairballs.

First Aid Recommendations for Coughing

Do not give any medication!

Over-the-counter and prescription medication for use in people can be dangerous to dogs and cats.

Keep the animal's stress to a minimum, and do not allow strenuous activity.

Contact your veterinarian for an appointment.

Skin Emergencies

Excessive Scratching

Skin allergies are common in dogs and less common in cats.

Excessive scratching is one of the first signs of allergies.

Excessive scratching is not typically an emergency unless the skin is scratched so hard that it is bleeding.

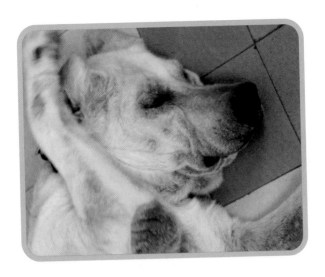

"Hot Spots"

A **hot spot** is a small area of irritation that can develop a topical, or surface, infection.

Most dogs will scratch at the site and cause more trauma to the skin.

The combination of skin trauma caused by scratching, the normal bacteria of the skin, and the protection provided by the animal's hair results in a vicious circle: scratching, continued infection, continued itching, scratching, and so on.

The topical infection looks moist and may be bleeding.

The affected area continues to spread, and your veterinarian's help is usually needed.

First Aid Recommendations for Skin Emergencies

Removing the hair with electric grooming clippers can help keep the infection from spreading.

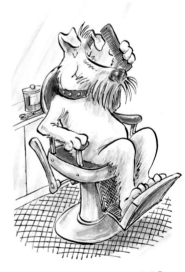

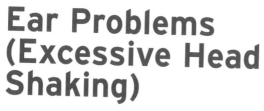

The hair will need to be clipped down to the level of the skin to be helpful.

Do not use any medication on the area!

Contact your veterinarian!

Some "hot spots" rapidly become so severe that a visit to the emergency clinic may be required.

NEVER use scissors to remove hair!

Ear Problems (Excessive Head Shaking)

Infections

Bacterial infections may develop in the ears of dogs and cats.

The inside of the ear is red.

There may be a tan discharge (pus) that could contain blood.

The dog or cat may shake its head excessively.

First Aid Recommendations for Ear Infections

Do not use any medication in the ear! Accidentally using medication containing just cortisone could make the infection worse. Contact your veterinarian!

144

Do not put petroleum jelly (Vaseline) or any other ointment in the ear.

Carefully wipe away any blood or other drainage from the inside or outside of the ear. Dogs and cats have a vertical (up-and-down) ear canal that leads to a horizontal (side-to-side) ear canal. People only have a horizontal ear canal. There is a slim chance of damaging the eardrum of a dog or cat.

Dogs and cats commonly use the hind legs to scratch their ears. Keeping the toenails of the hind legs cut short can help protect the ear from trauma.

Hematomas

Dogs with droopy ears that excessively shake the head can burst small blood vessels under the skin of the ear.

The build-up of blood from the broken vessels under the skin is called a **hematoma**.

Hematomas look like swelling of the ear. The swelling is caused by the build-up of blood under the skin.

Most hematomas require examination and treatment by your veterinarian.

First Aid Recommendations for Hematomas

Do not cut open the hematoma!

Improper treatment can make the hematoma worse or can cause infection under the skin.

Compress the ear if the dog scratches open the hematoma.

Excessive bleeding typically does not happen.

Limping

Weight-Bearing Limping

Injury to a leg can be minor, so the dog or cat will use the leg but sometimes will raise the leg during a step.

When standing, some dogs and cats will appear to touch only the toes on the ground, instead of the entire paw.

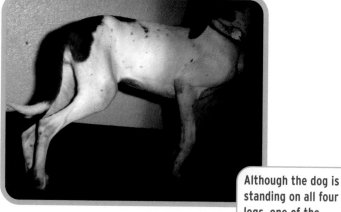

Although the dog is standing on all four legs, one of the hindlimbs is not placed entirely on the ground.

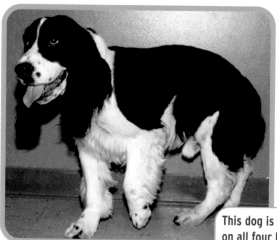

This dog is standing as if on all four legs, but one of the front legs is not on the ground at all.

Non-Weight-Bearing Limping

Injury to a leg can be major, so the dog or cat will not use the limb at all, either walking or standing.

Injury can happen to the bone, muscle, ligament, tendon, or capsule that surrounds the joints.

A physical examination and an x-ray study are needed to make the proper diagnosis and to choose the appropriate treatment.

First Aid Recommendations for Limping

Safety first!

Do not attempt to figure out if a bone is broken.

A muzzle may be required for transport of the injured animal to a veterinarian.

Less handling of the animal is usually better than attempting to use a board or a stretcher for transport.

Limping can have many causes besides a break in the bone. Using a **splint** is discouraged until a diagnosis can be made.

Worms

Puppies and Kittens

Intestinal worms are very common in puppies and kittens. In fact, most puppies and kittens either are born with worms or get worms early in life.

Diarrhea is a very common sign of worms, although bowel movements can appear to be normal.

Where We Stand

Annual examination of feces for worms is highly recommended for all dogs and cats, especially those that live outdoors or those that are allowed to roam large areas of farm and/or woods.

Occasionally, the bowel movements may contain worms (such as roundworms) that appear as white to brownish white strings that may or may not be moving.

- **Roundworms rarely cause life-threatening illness.**
- **However, ridding puppies and kittens of round- worms can help in removal of eggs from their en- vironment.**

Several types of worms such as hookworms and whip- worms are microscopic and cannot be seen with the naked eye.

- **Hookworms (in puppies and kittens) and whip- worms (in puppies only) can cause internal in- testinal bleeding that may or may not be seen in a bowel movement.**

Where We Stand

Giving over-the-counter medications to elimi- nate worms is not recommended. Many types of worms are not eliminated with these medications. Puppies or kittens with potentially life-threaten- ing loss of blood due to whipworms or hookworms will not be helped by these medications.

- **Life-threatening loss of blood can occur if worm infestation is not treated properly.**
- **Pale gums and extreme lethargy and depression (see Chapter 6: First Aid for Triage Level 1 Patients) can be signs of severe internal bleeding caused by worms.**

Tapeworms are the other type of worm that can be seen in the bowel movement.

- **Tapeworms develop after a puppy or kitten eats a flea.**

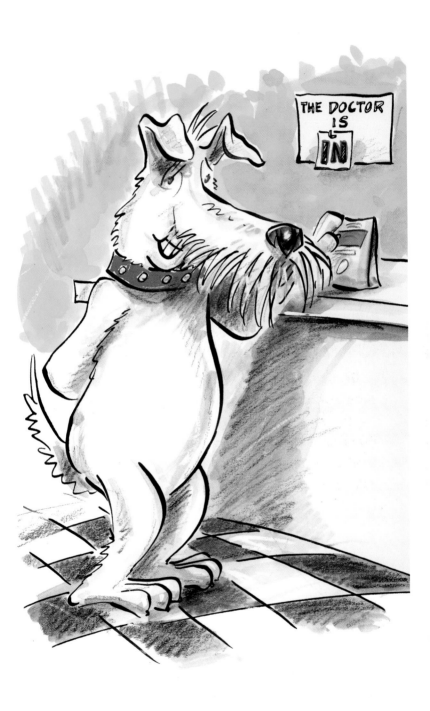

149

- Tapeworms may appear similar to roundworms, except that tapeworms have segments.
- Tapeworms rarely cause life-threatening illness.
- A diagnosis of tapeworms usually means a need for adequate flea control.

Adult Dogs and Cats

Adult dogs can become infected with worms such as hookworms, whipworms (in dogs only), and tapeworms. Roundworms in adult 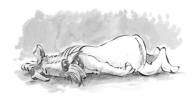 dogs and cats are uncommon.

Hookworms and whipworms are in the environment.

- An outdoor dog kennel in an area with dirt, grass, or gravel is a perfect environment for ongoing worm infestations.
- Diarrhea, especially containing blood, is a common sign of hookworm or whipworm infestation.
- Bowel movements can be normal.

Tapeworms are very common in adult dogs and cats.

- Tapeworms are transmitted to dogs and cats by one of two methods:
  Eating an adult flea
  Eating the intestines of wild animals (mice, rats)
- Tapeworms are generally harmless.
- Tapeworms may appear as long strands of segments (similar in appearance to roundworms) or as single, dried segments that look like grains of rice.

First Aid Recommendations for Worms

Seeing worms in a normal bowel movement of a dog or cat is not an emergency.

Sluggishness, depression, and pale gums in a puppy or kitten with or without blood in the bowel movement could mean a serious, life-threatening infestation of intestinal worms (hookworms or whipworms).

Over-the-counter deworming medication does not work to eliminate several types of worms.

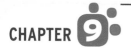

PET FIRST AID KIT

The items we suggest that you keep in this first aid kit are intended to keep the first aid provider safe while quickly getting the animal to a veterinarian.

The list of items can be long! Pet first aid kits can be put together in two different versions. The basic version consists of those items considered the bare essentials—ones that all first aid providers could easily keep on hand or in their vehicles. The second, more extensive version contains additional items for those first aid providers who work with rescue organizations.

Bare Essentials First Aid Kit

- Medium and large thick blankets or towels (A)
- Plywood or other section of wood (B)
- Medium to large cardboard box (C)
- Tape: electrical, duct, or packaging (D)
- Rope to use as muzzle (E)
- Rope leash (F)
- Newspaper to use for splints (G)

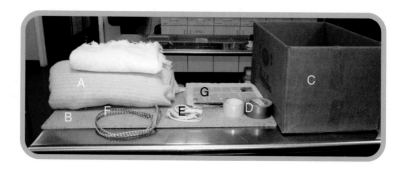

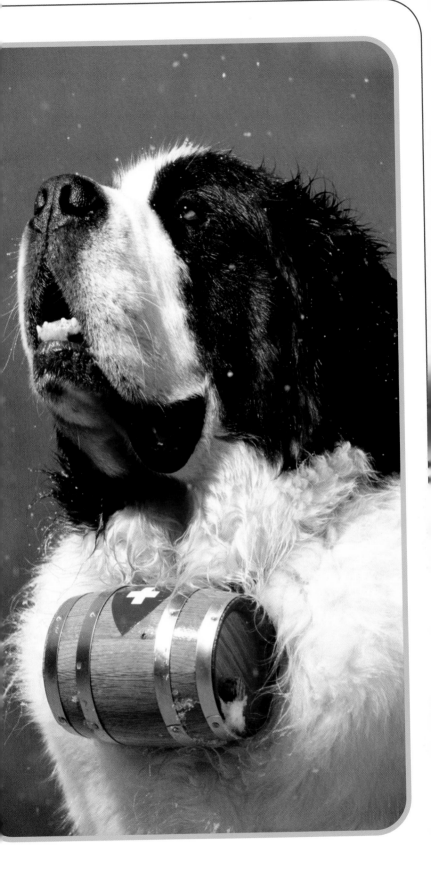

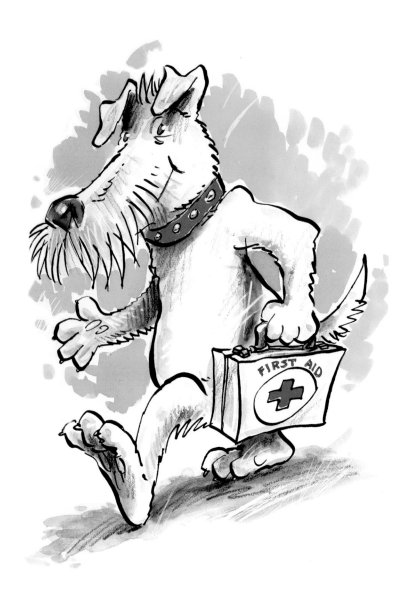

Extensive First Aid Kit

- All items from the bare essentials first aid kit (A)
- Fish net or commercially made net device to capture small dogs and cats (B)
- Commercially made muzzles for small, medium, and large dogs (C)
- Several small towels for compressing bleeding wounds (D)
- 4 × 4 gauze sponges and/or laparotomy sponges (E)
- Battery-operated clippers to clip hair from wounds (F)
- Commercially made stretcher (G)

154

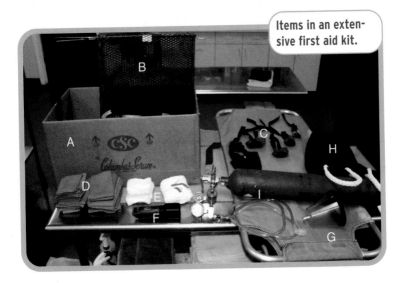

Items in an extensive first aid kit.

- Commercially made slings (H)
- Portable oxygen tank with tube, mask, and flow-by oxygen apparatus (I) (CAUTION: Oxygen tanks are under pressure, and oxygen causes combustion. Oxygen tanks require special handling, and permits may be required to carry an oxygen tank in your vehicle. Please check with the local authorities in your area. Do not carry oxygen tanks without proper permission.)

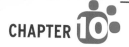

FINAL RECOMMENDATIONS

The following passages from the previous chapters are intended to highlight the most important parts of first aid.

Safety of the First Aid Provider

The first aid provider's safety is essential in order to help ill and injured animals.

The Family Pet

The gentlest family pet could hurt the pet owner if it is ill or injured. Remember, if you become injured by a bite or scratch, you may not be able to help your pet.

The Stray Animal

Injured stray animals may not be used to people and may become aggressive, in addition to being injured. Use appropriate restraint when helping stray animals. The best restraint may be as little restraint as possible.

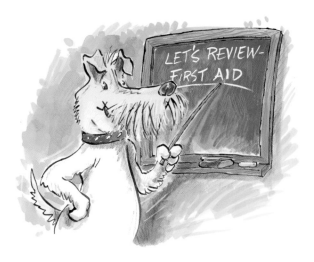

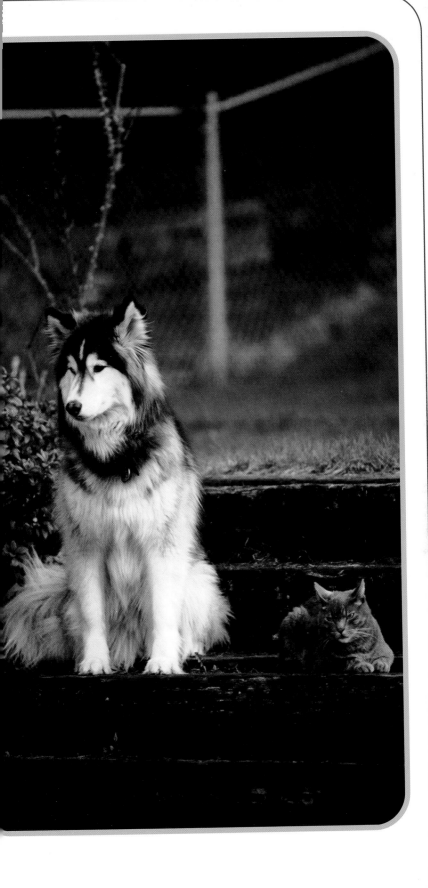

Triage

Deciding on the level of triage will help establish what level of first aid is needed.

Triage Level 1

- Patients are in critical condition and may survive if simple lifesaving steps are used.

- Pet owners can use the general guidelines of triage to decide what kind of first aid an ill or injured dog and cat immediately needs.

- First aid for triage level 1 patients may include basic life support CPCR techniques.

Triage Level 2

- Patients are likely to survive if simple care is given within hours.

- First aid providers may be tempted to medicate and treat animals themselves.

- Remember that patients in triage level 2 can quickly become triage level 1 patients if first aid and transport to a veterinarian are delayed.

Triage Level 3

- Patients have minor injuries that can wait for care while other, more critical patients are helped.

- First aid providers may be strongly tempted to hold off on treatment and medicate these animals themselves.

- Remember that any triage level 2 or 3 patient can quickly progress to a more serious category.

- Getting the animal to a veterinarian is a much better option than treating and medicating the pet at home, without a veterinarian's recommendations.

ABC Principle

These are the essentials of cardiopulmonary cerebral resuscitation (CPCR) and first aid for triage level 1 patients.

Alertness and Airway

- Understand and be familiar with the normal level of alertness and normal breathing sounds coming from the airway. There should be no airway sounds unless the dog is a breed that is apt to have noisy breathing.

- Depression or sluggishness is a common sign of problems.

- A dog or cat that you can hear breathing may be having a serious upper airway problem.

Breathing

- Understand and be familiar with normal breathing rates and breathing effort in dogs and cats.

- Breathing in (inspiration) is active, and breathing out (expiration) is passive (not requiring work from the animal).

- Exaggerated breathing in or out is not normal.

- High or low breathing rates are normal.

Circulation

- Understand and be familiar with dog and cat blood circulation parameters, including gum color, heart and pulse rate, and capillary refill time (CRT).

- A change in one aspect of circulation usually means that other aspects have changed as well.

RAP Principle

RAP is an alternative to the ABCs of CPCR, based on the same basic ideas in life support:

- **Respiration**
- **Alertness**
- **Perfusion**

Do No Harm

Restraint

- **Understand that proper restraint may be less restraint.**
- **Keep the animal's stress to a minimum at all times!**
- **Avoid being injured!**
- **Safe and quick transport depends on proper restraint.**

Self-medication

- Giving animals human medications is always a dangerous decision.
- Self-medication could be life-threatening or fatal!
- Do not self-medicate!

Transport

- The ability to quickly and safely transport a dog or cat to a veterinarian is the most important part of first aid.
- Understand the various ways to use adequate (but minimal) restraint and quick, safe transport.

Glossary

ABC principle   assessment of <u>a</u>lertness and <u>a</u>irway, <u>b</u>reathing, and <u>c</u>irculation

abdominal distention   an enlargement of the abdominal cavity

advanced life support (ALS)   a technique directed at restoring blood flow to the brain, as well as providing basic resuscitation measures

anaphylaxis   serious allergic reaction that causes shock and collapse

aspiration pneumonia   pneumonia that is caused by inhaling of stomach contents that were produced by vomiting or regurgitation

asthma   a condition in which the small airway tubes in the lungs are inflamed and air cannot be transported to or from the lungs

bloat   a condition in which the stomach is larger than normal, although it remains in its normal position

blunt trauma   trauma in which the skin or soft tissue has not been broken or penetrated, but may involve internal bleeding

brachycephalic   flat-faced; dogs with flat faces include the Bulldog, Boston Terrier, and Pug

bronchitis   inflammation and swelling of the airways (bronchi)

capillary refill time   the time it takes for the blanched (white) gums to return to normal color

cardiac arrest   a condition in which the coronary arteries become blocked, the heart beats become irregular, and heart muscles die from lack of oxygen (also called myocardial infarction or heart attack)

cardiomyopathy   failure of the heart muscle to pump properly

cardiopulmonary function   functions of the heart and the lungs, taken together

cardiopulmonary resuscitation (CPR)   a technique to revive (resuscitate) people or animals from unconsciousness or apparent death

cardiopulmonary-cerebral resuscitation (CPCR)   restoration of normal heart, lung, and brain function

circulation parameters   a measure of heart rate and rhythm, pulse rate and strength, and the coordination of heart and pulse rates

colitis   inflammation of the colon

congestive heart failure   breathing problems in dogs and cats that are a result of heart failure

do no harm   the goal in an emergency setting is to provide aid but to do no harm.

expiration   breathing out

first aid   basic treatment techniques applied at the scene of an accident or used when alarming changes in behavior or appearance suggest severe illness

fungal pneumonia   pneumonia that is caused by fungal organisms found in soil

heat exhaustion   rise in an animal's body temperature to between 103 and 105 degrees F when active or exercising in warm or hot outside (environmental) temperatures

heatstroke   rise in an animal's body temperature to higher than 105 degrees F when active or exercising in warm or hot outside (environmental) temperatures

Heimlich maneuver   method of dislodging food or other material from the throat of a choking victim

hematoma   a collection of blood under the skin from broken blood vessels due to trauma

hobble   something used to fasten an animal's legs together to prevent it from straying

hot spot   a small area of skin irritation, often very inflamed, that can develop a surface infection

hypothermia   body temperature lower than normal

inspiration   breathing in

paraphimosis   prolonged engorgement of the penis, potentially causing tissue to die as a result of lack of blood flow

penetrating trauma trauma in which the skin or soft tissue has been broken or penetrated

pericardial effusion filling of the sac around the heart with fluid

prepuce outer covering of the penis

prolapse condition in which the inside part of the large intestine (rectum) can begin exiting the anus in dogs and cats that are straining to defecate or urinate

RAP principle assessment of respiration, alertness, and perfusion (blood circulation)

respiratory arrest a total inability to continue breathing

reverse sneezing vigorous and extremely loud snorting sounds that happen rapidly together; unlike a regular sneeze, the efforts are inward rather than outward

seizure chaotic release of brain waves

shock a life-threatening condition of inadequate blood flow to the body's organs

splints temporary tools used to stabilize the two or more parts of a broken bone

torsion condition in which the stomach enlarges and twists around on itself

triage the process of prioritizing sick or injured people or animals for treatment according to the seriousness of the condition or injury

triage level 2 category for ill or injured patients who usually survive if they receive simple care within a few hours

triage level 3 category for patients who have minor injuries or illnesses that can wait for treatment while other, more critically ill or injured patients receive needed care

vestibular nerve a nerve linked to the ear that helps animals keep their normal balance

Credits

Page 23   Nelson RW, Couto CG: *Small Animal Internal Medicine*, ed 3, St Louis, 2003, Mosby.

Page 25 *(bottom)*   Kittleson MD, Kienle RD: *Small Animal Cardiovascular Medicine*, St Louis, 1998, Mosby.

Page 101   Johnston SD, Root Kustritz MV, Olson PNS: *Canine and Feline Theriogenology*, Philadelphia, 2001, Saunders.

Page 109   Courtesy Doug Mader.

Page 123   Battaglia A: *Small Animal Emergency and Critical Care*, St Louis, 2001, Mosby.

Page 136   McCarthy T: *Veterinary Endoscopy for the Small Animal Practitioner,* St Louis, 2005, Elsevier.

Page 138   King L: *Textbook of Respiratory Disease in Dogs and Cats*, St Louis, 2004, Elsevier.

Page 141   Kealy JK, McAllister H: *Diagnostic Radiology and Ultrasonography of the Dog and Cat*, ed 4, St Louis, 2005, Elsevier.

Page 143   Gotthelf L: *Small Animal Ear Diseases*, ed 2, St Louis, 2005, Elsevier.

Page 144   Medleau L, Hnilica K: *Small Animal Dermatology*, St Louis, 2001, Mosby.

Index

A
ABC principle, 20, 43-47, 159
Abdomen in breathing difficulty, 48
Abdominal distention, 78-81
Abnormal airway, 23
Abnormal alertness, 20-22
Abnormal behavior, 20-22
Accident, vehicle, 63-64
Acetaminophen
  as harmful, 33
  poisoning with, 26
  toxic in cats, 84-85
Advanced life support (ALS), 47
Advil, 85
Airway, 159
  abnormal, 23
  in basic life support, 43
  inflammation of, 59-60
  normal, 8-10
Alertness, 159
  abnormal, 20-22
  normal, 6
  in shock, 62
Allergic reaction, 115
Allergy, skin, 142-144
ALS (advanced life support), 47
Anaphylactic reaction, 114-115
Ant, tick, flea, and insect granule poisoning, 90
Antiarrhythmic drug, 87
Antidepressant, 86
Antidote
  for antifreeze poisoning, 88
  vitamin K as, 89
Antifreeze poisoning, 87-89
Antihypertensive drug, 86-87
Antiinflammatory drug, toxicity of, 85, 86
Arrest
  death and, 42
  respiratory versus cardiac, 42-43
Arrow wound, 69
Artificial circulation, 45-47
Aspiration pneumonia, 60
Aspirin, 83-84, 84-85
Asthma in cats, 59
Attention deficit hyperactivity disorder drug, 86
Australian Shepherd
  breathing rate in, 10
  heart rate in, 12
Azalea toxicity, 92

B

Bacterial pneumonia, 60
Balance, loss of, 128-129
Bandage, 72-74
Basic life support (BLS)
  airway in, 43
  breathing in, 44-45
  circulation in, 45-47
Bassett Hound
  abdominal distention in, 78-81
  pulse in, 14, 15
Behavior
  abnormal, 20-22
  normal, 6
Bile, aspiration of, 60
Birth
  care after, 103-104
  difficult, 100-104
  problems after, 105-106
  umbilical cord care after, 104
Birth canal, 100
Bite, snake, 108-110
Black mucous membrane, 16, 17
Bladder stone, 95
Blanket as restraint, 36
Bleeding
  bandages for, 72-73
  from rat and mouse bait poisoning, 89
Blinking, excessive, 116
Bloat, 79-81
Blockage, urinary, 95-96
Blood
  in bowel movement, 127-128
  circulation of, 10-19
  external bleeding and, 72
  shock and, 62
  sneezing and, 134, 136
  in urine, 127
  from vulva, 130-131
Blood cells, decrease in, 25
Blood pressure medication, 86-87
Blood sugar, low, 99-100
Blow-by oxygen for cat, 58, 61
BLS (basic life support), 45-47
Blue mucous membranes, 25
Blunt trauma
  from being caught in furniture, 65
  from being stepped on, 65
  dryer causing, 65
  fall causing, 64-65
  from fight, 70-72
  first aid for, 66-68
  impact from object causing, 65-66
  from motor vehicle, 63-64